Aromatherapy for Beginners

The Ultimate Guide to Relieve your Pain, Improve your Health and Relax your Mind using Aromatherapy and Essential Oils

Jane Moore

All Rights Reserved. No part of this publication may be reproduced in any form or by ay means, including scanning, photocopying, or otherwise without prior written permission of the copyright holder. Copyright © 2015

Contents

Introduction

What is Aromatherapy?

    What is the Difference Between Aromatherapy and Essential Oil Therapy?
    Can Aromatherapy Get Rid of My Pain, Reduce My Stress or Cure Me?
    How Will Aromatherapy and Essential Oils Benefit Me?
    8 Things You Should Know About Aromatherapy

Understanding Essential Oils

    The Chemical Makeup of Essential Oils - Constituents
    Are There Standards Used to Test Essential Oils?
    How Essential Oils Are Extracted
    3 Aromatherapy Models
    The 2 Main Methods of Using Essential Oils
    10 Essential Oil Safety Tips You Should be Aware Of
    How do I Know Which Company to Buy my Essential Oils From?
    What Should I Look For in the Bottling?

9 Ways You Can Use Essential Oils

1. Massage
2. Bath
3. Inhale Using a Tissue
4. Steam Inhalation
5. Insect Repellent
6. Freshen Your Home
7. Air Freshener
8. Personal Hygiene
9. Medicinal

Understanding Carrier Oils

    How to Store Your Carrier Oils

12 Essential Oils That Should be in Every Home

1. Bergamot
2. Clary Sage
3. Eucalyptus
4. Frankincense
5. Geranium
6. Lavender
7. Lemon
8. Oregano
9. Peppermint
10. Sandalwood
11. Tea Tree
12. Ylang Ylang

How to Blend Your Essential Oils

Blending Oils Based on Their Aroma

Understanding Essential Oil Notes

5 Things You Should Know About Blending Essential Oils

How to Create Your Own First Aid Kit With Essential Oils

Wound Healing With Essential Oils

Treat Nausea and Vomiting With Essential Oils

Reduce Jet Leg with Essential Oils

Treating Minor Aches and Pain with Essential Oils

Ease Muscle Spasms with Essential Oils

Treat Bee Stings and Bites with Essential Oils

Treat Minor Burns with Essential Oils

Treat Sunburn with Essential Oils

Wrapping it All Up

Calming Emotions Using Essential Oils

40 Aromatherapy Recipes You Can Make at Home

1. Bath Salts Recipe

2. Homemade Lotion Recipe
3. Massage Oil Recipe – 4 Options
4. Aromatherapy Bath Oil Recipe
5. Peppermint Rosemary Shampoo
6. Hair Conditioner
7. Acne Recipe
8. Sugar Facial and Body Scrub
9. Cuticle Oil
10. Rose Oil Aphrodisiac

Aromatherapy Perfume Recipes

11. Perfume Recipe
12. Alcohol or Water Base Perfume Recipe
13. Carrier Oil Base Perfume Recipe
14. Cologne Recipe
15. Body Splash Recipe

Aromatherapy Recipes for Around Your House

16. Aromatherapy Room Mister Air Fresheners
17. Aromatherapy Essential Oil Diffuser Blends – Mood Setters
18. Aromatherapy Essential Oil Diffuser Blends – Therapeutic
19. Aromatherapy Essential Oil Diffusion for Gratitude

Recipes for Therapeutic Aromatherapy

Preparing Your Essential Oils

20. Recipes to Relieve Anger
21. Recipes to Calm Anxiety
22. Recipes to Increase Confidence
23. Recipes to Calm and Relax
24. Recipes to Ease Depression
25. Recipes to Increase Energy
26. Recipe to Reduce Menstrual Cramps
27. Recipe to Reduce the Symptoms For Cold & Flu
28. Recipe for Vaginal Dryness

29. Recipe to Fight Germs
30. Recipe to Stop Snoring
31. Recipe to Make Your Own "Vapor-Rub"
32. Recipe for Cough Syrup
33. Recipe for Ear Infection

Natural Home Care Recipes

34. Recipe for Natural Laundry Detergent
35. Recipe for Homemade Bleach
36. Recipe for Citrus All-Purpose Cleaner
37. Recipe for Fabric Softener
38. Recipe to Control Pet Odor
39. Recipe for Glass Cleaner
40. Recipe for Dish Soap

Conclusion

Introduction

Welcome – I'm happy to help you explore your interest in aromatherapy. You may already have a bit of knowledge or perhaps you have simply heard others talking about aromatherapy.

This book is designed for the beginner who wants to get an understanding of aromatherapy, how it can improve your health, relax your mind and relieve your pain.

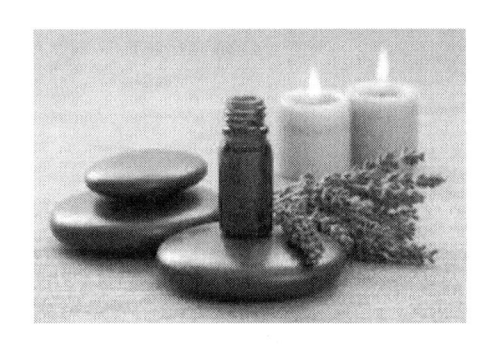

Aromatherapy can benefits you both psychological and physically. You can use aromatherapy a number of ways, from personal use to around your home, and of course medicinally. Using aromatherapy around the home can help to create a more relaxed and healthy mind – a more balanced mind.

In this book, you will learn about many of the essential oils available and using them therapeutically. You will also learn about the different carrier oils and choosing the best one for your recipe. You will learn what the difference is between aromatherapy and essential oil therapy.

By the time you get through this easy to understand book, you will have tons of knowledge and be well equipped to begin to make your own aromatherapy recipes. While this book is written for beginners, it's definitely not limited to beginners. Even if you have a working knowledge of aromatherapy and essential oils, you'll find this book a valuable reference. Moreover, you can continue to use and enjoy the recipes for years to come, to help you with physical and mental ailments.

Are you ready? Let's get started.

What is Aromatherapy?

When you hear the word aromatherapy, what do you think of? Do you think of things that smell nice like potpourri, perfumes, scented candles or room diffusers? Actually, that's not what aromatherapy means at all.

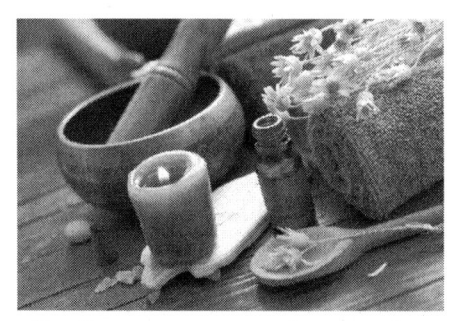

Aromatherapy isn't new. Essential oils have been used for thousands of year, although the term itself wasn't used until during the 20th century. Aromatherapy is simply the practice of using volatile plant oils for your mental, emotional and physical well-being. This includes the use of essential oils, which is the basis of aromatherapy.

Essential oils are a used in aromatherapy recipes, along with other natural ingredients that might include things like sea salts, herbs, clays, and vegetable oils. Since this is a book on aromatherapy, not only will we look at essential oils, I will cover a number of the other natural ingredients that are part of aromatherapy recipes.

When you use aromatherapy, it is best if you can keep this practice as holistic as possible. That is how you will derive the most benefits. Always choose the highest quality natural ingredients you can find and avoid using synthetic ingredients, which have no medicinal value.

What is the Difference Between Aromatherapy and Essential Oil Therapy?

There's often confusion over these two therapies, but actually they are the same thing.

Aromatherapy implies that all essential oils have a nice aroma or smell. However, that's a bit of a misnomer, since there are many essential oils that have very unpleasant smells. For example, valerian or German chamomile, do not appeal to most people.

Aromatherapy also implies that the only way that you can enjoy therapeutic benefit from the essential oils is to inhale or smell. That's also an incorrect belief.

There are many ways that you can benefit from using essential oils. Later on, I am going to look at these ways in detail.

Can Aromatherapy Get Rid of My Pain, Reduce My Stress or Cure Me?

If you were told that you can cure your disease, illness, or injury using just aromatherapy, you need to believe with at least a little skepticism. Essential oils can do so much! They can reduce even eliminate your pain, they can help you find emotional balance, they can be used to treat many different ailments and injuries. Like all holistic avenues of healing, they offer many great benefits, but they are not magic bullets.

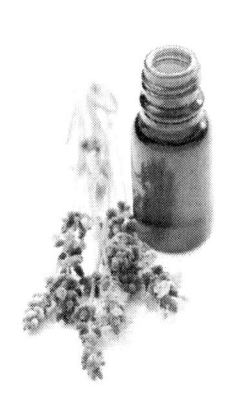

However, if you are realistic in your expectations of what aromatherapy can do for you, you'll be pleasantly surprised at just how great the benefits are.

Essential oils can be life changing and for anyone looking to live a healthier, cleaner life, free of toxins aromatherapy and essential oils help you achieve that goal

Aromatherapy can help relieve or eliminate symptoms that are caused by disease or illness, it can help to improve your mood, it can eliminate or reduce your stress temporarily and that's just a few of the benefits you can experience. I encourage you to read the entire book, so that you have a full understanding of how aromatherapy works and the important role therapeutic essential oils play in healing. That way you will get the maximum benefits.

Holistic aromatherapy is an excellent complementary alternative health choice. It is not designed to replace medical care, nor do I advocate that you do, but it nicely compliments those services and it can help to keep you healthy and full of vitality. It can speed up healing of injuries, help with pain, improve your emotional and mental well-being, and treat many ailments. In some cases, it is an excellent alternative to prescriptions or over the counter drugs.

Aromatherapy is terrific to eliminate common symptoms and ailments like indigestion, colds, cuts, inflammation, bruises, muscle stiffness, acne, arthritis, skin care, PMS, hair care, stress, insomnia, concentration, and the list goes on.

Aromatherapy can be very beneficial; however, common sense must prevail. Please do not let yourself fall victim to outrageous claims about what aromatherapy can do such as cure cancer. Using essential oils is a great way to help you become a healthier person, but it should not be your lifeline for a serious medical condition.

How Will Aromatherapy and Essential Oils Benefit Me?

There are so many benefits to using essential oils in aromatherapy; I couldn't possibly list them all, so I've chosen 8 of the main benefits.

1. **Essential oils are organic substances that come from plants.** Essential oils support bringing your body back into balance without the harmful side effects that pharmaceuticals cause. You need to make sure you are using therapeutic grade essential oils, because other grades can contain harmful chemicals.

2. **Essential oils are quick and easy to use.** During the day, you can wear your essential oils and at night, you can diffuse them. Use essential oils to balance and heal the mind, body and soul.

3. **Essential oils immediately penetrate the cell membranes and the skin.** They can instantly penetrate the blood and tissue. They cross the brain-blood barrier and reach limbic parts of the brain that are responsible for your emotions and moods, so they can be beneficial in handling stress, dealing with sadness or anger, and other emotions.

4. **Essential oil are high in antioxidants.** Antioxidants strengthen your body and work to help eliminate free radicals.

5. **Essential oil have oxygenating properties.** This allows them to transport nutrients right to the cells that are oxygen deprived.

6. **Essential oils soothe your muscles and joints.** Essential oils are excellent at helping with minor aches and pains.

7. **Essential oil will soothe your digestion.** When it comes to soothing digestion, peppermint is one of the most regarded herbs.

8. **Essential oil can provide you with green household products.** There is no need to use toxic chemical products in your home, when you can make everything you will ever need from essential oils combined with other natural ingredients.

8 Things You Should Know About Aromatherapy

1. Never purchase perfume oils for therapeutic use. They do not have the benefits that pure essential oils have.

2. Never store pure, undiluted essential oils in bottles that have a rubber stopper, because the rubber breaks down and ruins the oil.

3. You can store your blended essential oils in a carrier oil in a glass bottle with dropper top a couple of months.

4. Do not purchase oils unless you can be sure of the quality. Buy reputable brands of oils. It's one of the mistakes beginners make. They buy on price and don't get the quality.

5. Have fun and explore aromatherapy. Start with the recipes in this book.

6. Store all of your essential oils in dark glass bottles and in a cool, dark place.

7. Know the safety information associated with each essential oil you are going to use.

8. You should know whether an essential oil you are thinking of buying is organic, ethically farmed or wild-crafted. You also want to know what country the

essential oil originated from. It makes it easier when you are comparing suppliers to have all the information upfront.

Understanding Essential Oils

Essential oils come from the plant's true essence. Usually an essential oil is distilled using steam or water. It can be the leaves, flowers, stems, roots, bark or a combination of plant parts. Essential oils are generally clear, but some oils like patchouli, orange or lemongrass are amber in color.

Don't confuse therapeutic essential oils with fragrance oils, also called perfume oils, which contain synthetic chemicals and have no therapeutic value.

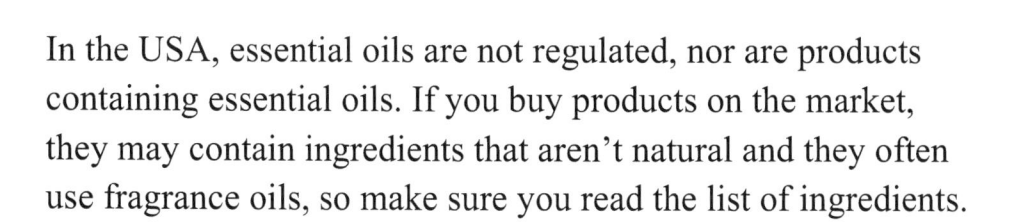

In the USA, essential oils are not regulated, nor are products containing essential oils. If you buy products on the market, they may contain ingredients that aren't natural and they often use fragrance oils, so make sure you read the list of ingredients.

Even when a product claims to be made from natural ingredients or made with essential oils, you still need to be cautious, because if the product doesn't say that it's made only from natural ingredients or essential oils it could contain a mix of natural and synthetic ingredients. A manufacturer needs to add only a few drops of essential oil and they are able to claim that product is 'made with essential oils,' even if all of the other ingredients are synthetic.

If you really want to be sure, you are using the highest quality therapeutic product, it's simple, make it yourself. In fact, later on I am going to give you tons of great recipes to get you started.

In most cases, you will dilute your essential oils with a carrier, before you apply it to your skin to be absorbed. With some oils, you'll get the therapeutic benefits through inhalation.

The quality and price of an essential oil depends on many different variables, such as where the essential oil originates from, the distiller's standards, the growing conditions, how much oil the plant produces, and how rare the plant is.

The Most Common Therapeutic Uses

- **Lavender** - Cuts, scrapes, minor burns, wound care, pain relief and insomnia
- **Basil** - Anti parasitic and insect repellent
- **Rosemary** - Anti-infective agent and stimulant
- **Bergamot** - Mild antidepressant and tonic
- **Eucalyptus** - Respiratory infections, colds and sinuses
- **German chamomile** - Inflammatory skin conditions
- **Ginger** - Nausea, vomiting and inflammation
- **Lemongrass** - Fungal infections
- **Peppermint** - Headaches, nausea, and fever
- **Tea Tree** - Viral, fungal and bacterial infections

The Chemical Makeup of Essential Oils - Constituents

There are two main constituent groups used to identify the chemistry of essential oils. They are **oxygenated compounds and hydrocarbons**. These two groups are divided into a number of sub-groups.

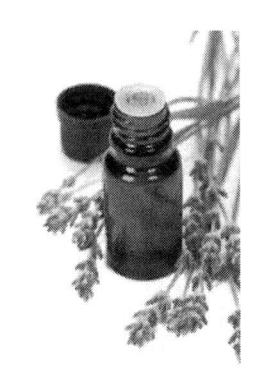

1. **Sesquiterpenes**

Sesquiterpenes erase bad information that is stored in your cellular memory. Nearly every essential oil has sesquiterpenes. Essential oils chemistry says that sesquiterpenes are the biggest group of terpenes known to exist in the animal and plant kingdom

Sesquiterpenes are larger than monoterpenes and they are less volatile, so you will find them commonly used as a fixative within the perfume industry. The half-life of viscous oils is longer and they blend well with the lighter and more volatile essential oils.

Examples of essential oils containing high levels of sesquiterpenes include myrrh, sandalwood and cedarwood.

2. **Monoterpenes**

All essential oils contain monoterpenes, which stop toxins from accumulating in your cells, and they restore your DNA so it has the correct information after sesquiterpenes and pheonlicshave complete their role. Monoterpenes enhance the therapeutic values of the essential oil's components and they are the part of the oil that creates balance.

Examples of essential oils containing high levels of monoterpenes include orange, balsam fir and grapefruit.

3. Phenolics

Phenolics stimulate your immune system and nervous system. They clean up the cell's receptor sites so that sesquiterpenes can erase any faulty information your cells are carrying. They have excellent antioxidant properties.

Examples of essential oils containing high levels of phenolics include tea tree, wintergreen and cloves.

4. Alcohols

Animal studies have shown that alcohols are resistant to oxidation and they can revert cells back to normal function.

Examples of essential oils containing high levels of alcohol include geranium, rose otto and rosewood.

5. Aldehydes

Aldehydes are behind all the lovely essential oils fragrance. They calm the nervous system and are known to relax and reduce stress.

Examples of essential oils containing aldehydes include lemongrass, cinnamon and bark.

6. Esters

Esters occur because of a reaction of an alcohol with an acid. These essential oils are the most calming, relaxing and balancing of the constituents. They are an antispasmodic and they regulate the nervous system.

Examples of essential oils containing high levels of esters include Roman chamomile, valerian and bergamot.

7. Ketones

Keytones are not as common as alcohols and monoterpenes. They have distinctive fragrances. They calm and sedate, stimulate cell regeneration and liquefy mucous.

Examples of essential oils containing high levels of ketyones include rosemary and cedar.

8. Oxides

Oxides come from other compounds such as terpenes or alcohols, which have been oxidized. They are expectorants and they can be somewhat stimulating. Eucalyptol is the most common essential oil in the oxide family with many different species.

Examples of essential oils with oxides include eucalyptus and rosemary.

There are additional compound classes that essential oils can contain, but they are not the main ones and overall make up less than 20%. These are Ethers, Carboxylic Acids, Alkanes, Lactones, Furanoids and Coumarins.

While I have only touched on the chemistry makeup of essential oils, it shows that from the volatility, viscosity and medicinal properties, you can learn a lot about the chemistry profile can of the plant and the essential oil. Now when the safety information of an essential oil says avoid phenols you will understand what that means.

Because essential oils are made up of hundreds constituents and they come from a constantly changing environment, **no two batches of essential oils are ever going to be identical**. It's also why it is so hard to re-create them synthetically in the laboratory and why so many companies want to, so they can constantly offer a product that is exactly like a previous one. This is especially true in the perfume industry.

Are There Standards Used to Test Essential Oils?

In the United States there are **no** standards to test therapeutic grade essential oil. In fact, the FDA even has weak standards on even the labeling of oil, which means it is unreliable and deceptive.

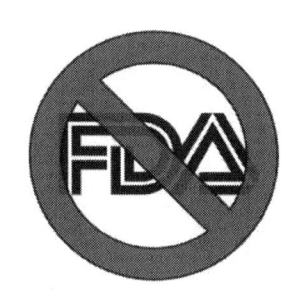

For example, an oil can be labeled generically thyme, without providing the chemotype or scientific name. What then are you really buying?

In Asian, Middle Eastern, and European cultures, where essential oils have been used for thousands of years, there are guidelines. The manufacturers who want to produce real therapeutic essential oils follow standards and test batches.

The AFNO and ISO standards provide the most reliable chemical constituent indicators to determine whether an essential oil is therapeutic. There is no organization in the world that regulates whether manufacturers are meeting the standards that are outlined. Testing is expensive so few companies actually carry it out.

How Essential Oils Are Extracted

There are different methods used to extract essential oils. The extraction process plays a role in defining whether an essential oil is therapeutic grade, aromatherapy grade or perfume grade.

Distillation and carbon-dioxide extraction methods use solvents and chemicals in a commercially manufactured processes to speed up the distillation process. The process is far less expensive, but the oils are changed.

These oils will have absorbed some of the solvent, so if you are using them for therapeutic use, it can pose a health risk. 98% of essential oils are manufactured this way including perfume quality oils.

Distillation using steam is done at very low temperatures so that the quality of the oil and the therapeutic values are maintained. This is a very slow process.

The distillation temperatures, type of condenser used and length of time the oil is distilled for all play a huge role in the oils quality.

Producing therapeutic grade oils is incredibly expensive. You need hundreds of pounds of plant to make a just one pound of therapeutic essential oil. For example, 60 roses will make a single drop of therapeutic rose oil. Yes **one drop**! It takes much less plant material to make perfume or synthetic grade oils.

Therapeutic oils are also incredibly expensive to produce and they take a long time. The cost alone can be a deterrent to companies. I encourage you to use therapeutic grade essential oils for everything you create.

3 Aromatherapy Models

There are 3 aromatherapy models that are used.
1. The German Model
2. The British Model
3. The French Models

Each of these models has a different way of applying essential oils to the body and they each approach the safety of essential oils differently.

The German Aromatherapy Model
The emphasizes is on the inhalation of essential oils. Research has confirmed that just inhaling the oils can be beneficial emotionally and physically. This model alone is very effective.

The British Aromatherapy Model
This model is very conservative and a high level of dilution is supported. The British tend to put too much emphasis on the safety of essential oils but not enough emphasis on using therapeutic grade oils.

The French Aromatherapy Model
This model is very proactive and they support applying essential oils undiluted to the skin. They also support the use of essential oils internally, in the form of vaginal and rectal implants.

Essential oils safety is never compromised. Those essential oils where it is critical that they be diluted are diluted. As well, those essential oils that should not be used internally are not used internally.

The French rely on solid scientific studies that focus on using therapeutic grade essential oils. There really aren't safety concerns if you use an essential oil that is therapeutic quality. The problem is that the majority of oils on the market are adulterated oils.

The United States does not use just one method and there is no US school of thought on aromatherapy and essential oils. It seems the US and Canada are more or less, just following a mixture of existing models and protocols.

I am talking about these three models because at some point you will likely come across information that's conflicting and this will help you to understand why that is happening.

The 2 Main Methods of Using Essential Oils

Inhaling Essential Oils

The inhalation of essential oils have mental and physical benefits. The aroma of the essential oil stimulates your brain to generate a specific reaction and when it is inhaled into your lungs, the active chemicals provide therapeutic benefits. For example, you inhale eucalyptus essential oil to help ease your congestion.

You need to make sure that you are always using essential oils in a safe manner and in the manner they are supposed to be used, so that you can enjoy the benefits and not experience any negative effects. Remember essential oils are medicinal and should be treated as such.

Essential Oils Applied to the Skin

When you apply essential oils to your skin, they are absorbed into your bloodstream providing numerous health benefits. Because essential oils are concentrated they are very powerful, which is why seldom are they applied directly to the skin without first diluting with a carrier oil such as sweet almond oil, grapeseed oil or apricot kernel oil. I am going to go into detail on this a little later.

10 Essential Oil Safety Tips You Should be Aware Of

Essential oils are medicines, but sometimes users forget this and don't take appropriate action. Some safety information you should have:

1. **Always dilute the essential oils before you apply it to your skin.** The odd time, a practitioner or experienced user might apply a pure essential oil to the skin, but as a beginner, you should never do this unless a recipe instructs you to. If you are given no direction, assume it needs to be diluted with a carrier oil and do so before you apply the essential oil to your skin.

2. **Some essential oils are photosensitive.** These particular essential oils can cause irritation, inflammation, redness, blistering and/or burning if you apply them to the skin and then they are exposed to UVA/UVB rays. If an oil is phototoxic make sure that you stay out of the sun when you are using it.

3. **Allergic reactions or sensitivities occur occasionally.** The first time you apply an essential oil topically, do a skin patch test and wait a full 24-hours. While allergies and sensitivities are rare they do occur.

4. **Prior to using any essential oils talk to your doctor** if you have epilepsy, asthma, are pregnant, are nursing or have other health conditions. Research and review all safety precautions associated with each essential oil that you use, medications that you take and conditions you might have.

5. **Some essential oils should be used only by experienced users or trained professionals.** Wormwood, onion, camphor, pennyroyal, horseradish, bitter almond, wintergreen, etc. are examples of some of the essential oils that should be used only by professional users.

6. **Do not use essential oils on children** without knowing everything about the essential oil and its use on children. Treat essential oils the same way you treat all medications that are potentially poisonous in the hands of children. Use only as directed for children, and don't use on children if the oil says not to.

7. **Use the smallest amount of essential oil possible.** Essential oils are highly concentrated, so start with the smallest amount and increase slowly. For example, if 1-2 drops are called for, start with one drop, if that doesn't work go to two drops, but don't increase past that. High doses are wasteful and not necessary.

8. **Do not take essential oils internally.** A qualified practitioner is the only one who should be telling you to take an essential oil internally after a detailed

consultation with you. It is not advisable for you to take this on yourself.

9. **Store essential oils away from fire hazards.** Essential oils are highly flammable.

10. **If you are pregnant** do not use clary sage essential oil, marjoram essential oil or rosemary essential oil. There is a documented case that these oils have caused a miscarriage. If you are pregnant it is important that you are careful when using any essential oils. The best course of action would be to consult with your doctor or naturopath.

How do I Know Which Company to Buy my Essential Oils From?

You can make your own recipes, but ultimately, you are going to have to buy your therapeutic grade essential oils from somewhere. So how do you pick? What do you look for in a company?

There are several things to consider when you are looking for a company that supplies quality therapeutic grade essential oils.

1. A company that either grows or buys organic plant material to distill.
2. A company that doesn't distill using plants that have been treated or exposed to pesticides, fertilizers or chemicals.
3. A company who is involved in the process of harvesting and distilling, so that they can ensure quality control.
4. A company who is environmentally conscious and does not over harvest rare plants or trees, and who works with agencies to save endangered species.
5. A company whose primary method of extraction is steam distillation.
6. A company that meets or exceeds AFNOR standards.

What Should I Look For in the Bottling?

Buying an essential oil that has no details written on it is kind of like stumbling down a street in the middle of the night wearing a blindfold. You have no idea where you are going but you know that it's likely not going to end well. Using unmarked oils poses the same kinds of risks. You might not get any therapeutic value out of the oil and so you will have wasted your money, and it could actually pose a health risk.

Here are some things to look for:

- Oils should be packaged in an amber, violet or cobalt glass battle in order to preserve the purity of the oil.
- Oils should be properly sealed
- Oil bottles should have an orifice reducer.
- On the bottle should it should state the oil is 100% pure therapeutic grade essential oil.
- The oils volume should be clearly displayed. For example, 5 ml.
- Is should have the plants common name.
- The bottle should have the scientific name.
- Is should list the chemotype if applicable
- It should list instructions for use.
- It should list safety information.
- If there is a carrier oil it should be listed.
- If it is a blend everything should be listed.

There are reputable companies that provide consumers with therapeutic grade essential oils. Now that you know what to look for, you should have no trouble seeking them out.

9 Ways You Can Use Essential Oils

Using essential oils is easy and fun, and of course, therapeutic. There are many different ways that you can implement aromatherapy into your life and get the benefits it has to offer. Let's look at a few of the different ways that you can use essential oils.

1. Massage

Add 30-50 drops of your favorite essential oil to 2 ounces of carrier oil and massage on your body or give your partner a massage. How many drops will depend on the essential oil you are using and your scent preference – strong, medium, light. Keep oils away from your eyes and genitals. Always read the safety data for any essential oil or essential oil blend you choose to use.

2. Bath

Add 10-20 drops of essential oil to 1 ounce of carrier oil. Blend and then add it to your bath water. Swirl it in the water to ensure it is well mixed before you get into the bath. The number of essential oil drops you need is determined based on the essential oil and the benefit you are looking for.

3. Inhale Using a Tissue

A quick and easy way to get the benefits is to inhale an essential oil. Put 2 or 3 drops of essential oil on a tissue and then hold the tissue 1-2 inches from your nose and inhale. The first time you use an essential oil in this manner; start with one drop to determine if you have any sensitivity to the oil.

4. Steam Inhalation

Boil or microwave 3 cups of water. Pour the water into a glass or metal bowl. You should never use plastic as the heat can release toxins. Add 5-10 drops of essential oil to the water or whatever the amount the recipe calls for. Pine, eucalyptus and other similar oils need only 3-4 drops, because they can irritate your mucus membranes.

Choose your essential oil based on the therapeutic benefits you are looking for. For example, if you want to unplug the sinuses you might use eucalyptus oil.

Put a towel over your head, which should be 8 to 10 inches from the bowl and begin to inhale the steam. Inhale slowly breathing between inhales. Steam inhalation can really help with colds.

5. Insect Repellent

Lavender, rosemary, eucalyptus and citronella are all excellent insect repellents. There are others. Sprinkle 3 to 4 drops of essential oil on a cotton ball and then place the cotton balls near your doors and windows to keep the bugs away.

If you want to apply to your skin to keep insects at bay, grab an 8 ounce glass bottle and fill it half full with water that's been boiled, add 50 drops of your essential oil and then top up with witch hazel.

You can also use essential oils to protect your pets from fleas and ticks. However, some oils are not safe to apply directly on your pet, so it's best to play it safe and place the oils on the outside of their collar or on a scarf. They will still enjoy the protection, but without the risk.

6. Freshen Your Home

You can add a couple of drops of pure essential oil to your trash, your laundry, your drawers, the vacuum bag or just about anywhere else you like.

7. Air Freshener

Boil some water, 2 or 3 cups works well. Pour the water into a glass or metal bowl add 8 to 20 drops of essential oil. Place the bowl in your room of choice and enjoy the natural fragrance wafting through the room. The amount of oil will depend on how strong you want the aroma and which oils you are using, but on average 10 drops works well.

8. Personal Hygiene

You can use essential oils in homemade, facial cleansers, toners, lotions, body butters, shampoos, conditioners, perfumes, shower gels, soaps and much more.

9. Medicinal

Use essential oils to ease arthritis, relieve a cold, heal cold sores, eliminate a headache, prevent a migraine, cure fungus, cure infections and the list goes on. Essential oils offer excellent medicinal value. A reminder - you need to always use therapeutic grade oils.

Understanding Carrier Oils

Before I delve into the essential oils further, it's important for you to have a better understanding of carrier oils, because in the majority of cases, it is these carrier oils you are going to use to dilute your essential oils.

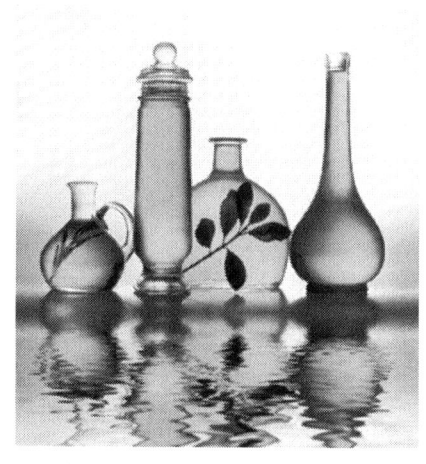

A carrier oil is a vegetable oil that is derived from the plant's fatty portion, which is generally the seeds, kernels, or nuts.

The carrier oil can be applied directly to your skin without diluting it. I use carrier oils to dilute essential oils so that they can be applied topically to the skin in the forms of lotions, creams, moisturizers, body oils, body butters, bath oils, lip balms and the list goes on.

Never use mineral oil or petroleum jelly as a carrier oil, because these are by-products of petroleum-based products so they are not considered natural and defeat your focus of a more natural, healthier and holistic lifestyle.

You will find mineral oil is in a large number of moisturizers that you buy. Companies love to use it, because it's so inexpensive for them to use. The trouble is that in addition to not being a natural option it can block toxins underneath the surface of the skin so they aren't able to leave your body. Long term this has the potential to increase your risk of cancer.

There are many common carrier oils that you can use. These are some of the most common:

1. Olive oil
2. Coconut oil
3. Sesame oil
4. Sunflower oil
5. Jojoba oil
6. Sweet almond oil
7. Grapeseed oil
8. Apricot kernel oil
9. Avocado oil
10. Peanut oil
11. Borage seed oil
12. Rose hip oil
13. Evening primrose oil
14. Hemp seed oil

Coconut oil, olive oil, sesame oil, sunflower oil and sweet almond oil are the most common carrier oils. Recipes will usually list a specific carrier oil to use, but in most cases, you can substitute carrier oils.

Sometimes there are specific properties to the carrier oil listed, which the recipe wants to incorporate for the maximum effect, so it pays to do a little research first. However, you will not wreck a recipe by substituting carrier oils, you just may not get the maximum benefits or it may change the texture or color.

How to Store Your Carrier Oils

Like your essential oils, to get the maximum life from your carrier oils you should store them in dark glass bottles with tight fitting tops. Store the bottle in a cool, dark location. If you will be using up a carrier oil long before its expected lifespan then it is not a important for the bottle to be dark in color, but you should always use glass bottles to store your carrier oils.

However, once you add essential oils to your carrier oil, you need to transfer the mixture to a dark glass bottle.

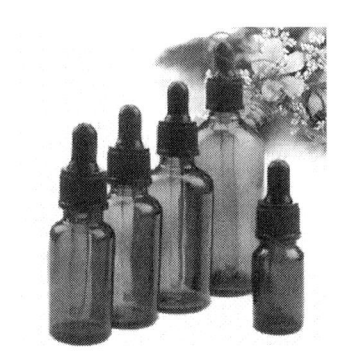

Most carrier oils can be stored in the refrigerator to help to maximize their lifespan. However, fragile oils like avocado oil and borage seed oil, should not be stored in the refrigerator.

When carrier oils are stored in the refrigerator they can solidify or turn cloudy, so you will need to return these oils to room temperature for some time before you use them, so that they can return to their liquid form.

12 Essential Oils That Should be in Every Home

You can invest in many different essential oils. In fact, there are so many that it can be a bit overwhelming trying to choose which ones to buy. If you start by making sure that you have these 12 essential oils in your home, you'll be in good shape.

1. Bergamot

Bergamot is an excellent essential oil to use on bacterial and viral infection since it has strong anti-viral and anti-inflammatory properties.

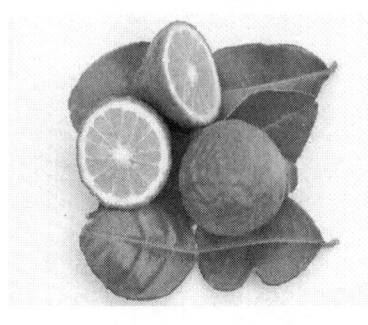

Just as it is a powerful antiseptic, it is also an excellent choice for inflammation in the body, such as that seen with arthritis. Bergamot can be used to treat the nervous system and it can be calming for emotions.

Use bergamot to:

- Relax muscle cramps (anti-spasmodic).
- Heal acne.
- Reduce lower back pain (anti-inflammatory).
- Stimulate circulation.
- Treat bacterial/viral infections of the mouth or nasal area.

- Balance your emotions.
- Help with anxiety and depression.
- Relieve the pain and swelling of insect bites/stings.
- Reduce the itch from allergies or bites/stings.
- Relax and calm the nervous system.
- Treat varicose veins.
- Treat minor cuts and scrapes. It will help you to heal faster and reduce scar tissue.

Important Note – In larger doses, bergamot is potentially unsafe in children. If you are pregnant or breast-feeding, or have diabetes, you should not use bergamot. Those with diabetes should not use bergamot as it may lower blood sugar levels. Stop using bergamot 2 weeks prior to any surgery.

2. Clary Sage

Clary sage balances and regulates the emotions. It can be helpful in combating insomnia and it is often used to clear the mind. Clary sage is an antibacterial, astringent and antiseptic.

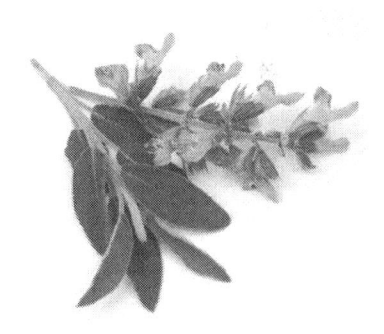

Use clary sage to:

- Treat acne.
- Lift depression.
- Make an excellent deodorant.

- Reduce gum disease.
- Reduce night sweats from menopause.
- Reduce varicose veins swelling.
- Improve sleep.
- Improve libido.
- Treat boils
- Treat infected pores.
- Treat bursitis.
- Improve your memory.

3. Eucalyptus

Eucalyptus is popular essential oil, especially when it comes to colds, respiratory infections and sinus problems. The invigorating aroma of eucalyptus is distinct and memorable. This is a very beneficial essential oil that should be in every home.

Use eucalyptus to:

- Disinfectant.
- Boost your immune system
- Treat respiratory ailments, including bronchitis.
- Treat sinus infections.
- Increase your alertness.
- Treat diarrhea.
- Treat bursitis, arthritis and tendinitis.

- Improve circulation.
- Treat bladder infections.
- Treat fungal infections.
- Improve your concentration.
- Relieve swelling, pain and itchiness from bug bites/stings.
- Relieve muscle spasms and lower back pain.
- Treat infected pores and boils.

Important Note – Never apply to your skin without first diluting. If you are pregnant or breast-feeding, do not use eucalyptus. 2 weeks prior to surgery stop using Eucalyptus.

4. Frankincense

Frankincense is an excellent essential oil when major healing is required. It has anti-tumor, anti-infection and anti-cancer properties.

Research has shown frankincense has the ability to penetrate the cell walls and restore damaged DNA.

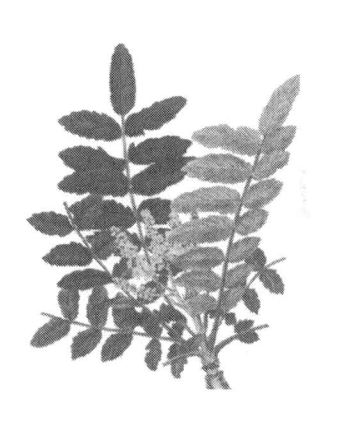

Frankincense is also a powerful choice for your spiritual well-being. It calms, centers and balances the emotional you.

Use frankincense to:

- Calm allergies.

- Focus and center you during times of trauma.
- Reduce the risk of tetanus.
- Reduce the signs of aging. Apply to your face and body.
- Reduce scars and stretch marks.
- Fade age spots
- Lift and tone your skin
- Reduce wrinkles.
- Center yourself before bed or before meditation.
- Boost your overall health (as a tonic).
- Freshen a room.
- Improve clarity.
- Clear a stuffy head.
- Help overcome depression.

5. Geranium

Geranium is a powerful antiseptic and astringent. It is also an excellent anti-inflammatory.

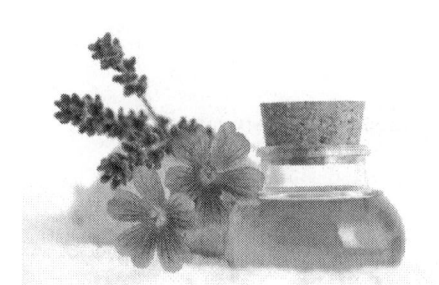

Use geranium to:

- Relieve headaches.
- Reduce symptoms of colds
- Relieve sore throats.
- Take care of your skin.
- Improve your memory.

- Treat emotional upset and mood swings
- Relieve anxiety.
- Reduce stress.
- Help with women's health issues.
- Treat varicose veins.
- Cure laryngitis.
- Treat athlete's foot.

6. Lavender

Lavender is one of the most commonly used essential oils that has been used for centuries. It is an antihistamine, anti-inflammatory, antidepressant, antimicrobial, anti-tumor and a pain reliever.

It also smells very nice. Lavender treats insomnia, yeast infections, allergies, cold sores, burns, anxiety, ringworm, dandruff, rash and more.

Use lavender to:

- Combat insomnia.
- Get rid of your dandruff.
- Exfoliate chapped lips.
- Spritz your linens.
- Add scent to your lotions and oils.
- Moisturize.

- To increase libido.
- Pamper your tired feet.
- Reduce the pain, swelling and itchiness of insect bites/stings.
- Relieve sunburn.
- Stop the itchiness of rashes.
- Reduce diaper rash.

Important Note – Some research indicates that for boys who have not yet reached puberty, there is a slight risk that lavender may disrupt normal hormones and cause boys to develop gynecomastia.

When Chloral Hydrate and other sedative medications are combined with lavender, it may increase drowsiness and sleepiness. 2 weeks prior to surgery, you should stop using lavender.

7. Lemon

Lemon essential oil is a powerful antiviral, antioxidant, antiseptic, antifungal and anti-cancer. Its uplifting aroma can put you in a good mood.

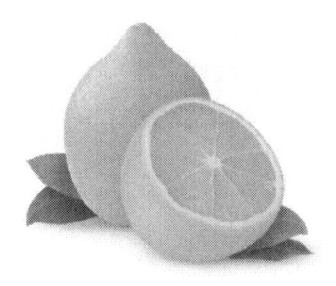

Use lemon to:

- Detox your body and energizes you. Just put a couple of drops in your water.
- Combat a sore throat.

- Kill germs. It's safer and more powerful than commercial hand sanitizers are.
- Improve your mood.
- Clean your fruit.
- Freshen your dish sponges.
- Use as a general cleaner to clean and disinfect your surfaces.
- Brighten your teeth.
- Heal cold sores.
- Dissolve your corns and calluses.

8. Oregano

Oregano boosts your immune response. It is an antifungal, anti-parasitic, antiviral and antibacterial.

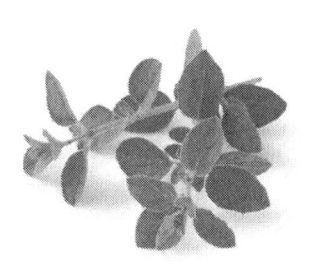

Use oregano to:

- Kill bedbugs, parasites and worms.
- Stop a sore throat.
- Treat eczema, psoriasis and other skin conditions.
- Prevent any infections and boost immunity.
- Rinse your vegetables and reduce food borne illnesses.
- Fight viruses.
- Reduce the symptoms of food poisoning.
- Clear your sinuses.
- Treat yeast infections.

- Keep your digestive tract healthy.

Important Note - Oregano is meant to be used short term. Infants, children, pregnant or nursing women, those with heart conditions or high blood pressure should not use therapeutic levels of oregano.

9. Peppermint

Peppermint is one of the most potent essential oils you will find. It is used for the digestive tract, motion sickness, heartburn and much more.

It has anti-inflammatory, antibacterial, anti-inflammatory, anti-carcinogenic and antiviral properties.

Use peppermint to:

- Invigorate you.
- Boost your energy.
- Relieve headaches.
- Treat nausea, indigestion, nausea, diarrhea, flatulence and other digestive conditions.
- Reduce fever.
- To reduce itchiness.
- Reduce arthritis inflammation and pain.
- Eliminate bad breath.

Important Note - Peppermint can cause allergic reactions in some. If you have achlorhydria, do not use enteric-coated peppermint oil. If you take medications that are broken down by the liver, peppermint can interfere and interact.

10. Sandalwood

Sandalwood has anti-inflammatory, antibacterial and antiseptic properties.

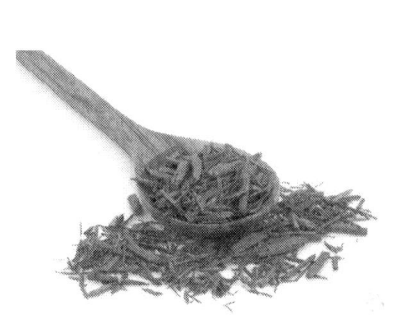

Use sandalwood to:

- Help scars to heal faster.
- Reduce lower back pain and arthritis pain.
- Reduce menstrual pain.
- Improve concentration.
- Reduces nervous tension, anxiety and stress.
- Increase libido.
- Help with insomnia.
- Relieve your cough.
- Help with skin conditions.
- Reduce the severity of menopausal night sweats and hot flashes.

Important Note - Do not use sandalwood if you are pregnant or breast-feeding.

11. Tea Tree

Tea tree is an essential oil is best known for its abilities to cure viral and bacterial infections.

Tea tree has antiseptic, antibacterial, anti-inflammatory, anti-fungal and antiviral properties. It has a very strong and distinct aroma.

You either like it or hate it, but even if you aren't fond of it, the benefits are worth tolerating it, and besides it usually grows on you over time.

Use tea tree to:

- Treat cuts and scrapes.
- Treat acne and oily skin.
- Treat sore throats and other mouth infections.
- Treat earaches.
- Treat cold & sinus problems.
- Provide cough relief.
- Heal and soothe sunburn.
- Remove skin tags and warts.
- Treats psoriasis and other skin conditions.
- Repel insects.

12. Ylang Ylang

Ylang Ylang has antidepressant, antiseborrhoeic, antiseptic and aphrodisiac properties.

Use ylang ylang to:

- Treat cuts, abrasions and burns so they heal faster and reduce infection.
- Stimulate your circulation.
- Help with anger and aggression.
- Treat acne.
- Increase your libido.
- Lower blood pressure.
- Help with nervous conditions.
- Promote healthy skin.
- Relax.

You should always treat therapeutic essential oils as medicines. I have noted some of the warnings, but this is by no means an inclusive list. If you are pregnant, nursing or have any health conditions before using any therapeutic essential oil or aromatherapy recipe you should talk to your doctor or naturopath.

In addition, if you are on any medications you should discuss with your doctor any possible interaction. Always discuss any concerns you have with your doctor or naturopath.

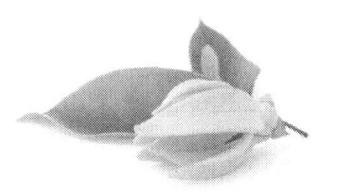

How to Blend Your Essential Oils

The practice of aromatherapy can be very rewarding, especially when you begin to create your own blends and make your own recipes. You can create blends for their therapeutic value along and you can create blends for the way that they smell. You can also create blends that combine the two.

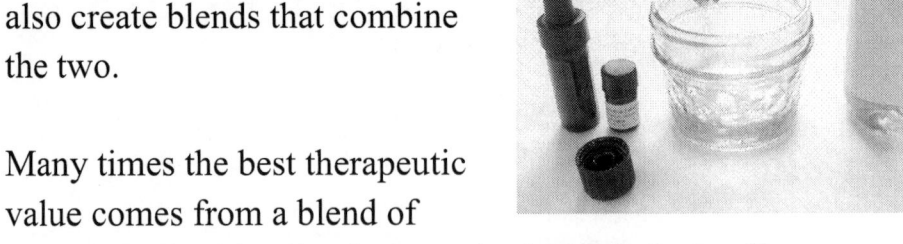

Many times the best therapeutic value comes from a blend of essential oils. Blending is not only therapeutic, it offers some very complex aromas that are very appealing.

When a specific blend of essential oils is created to deal with a certain therapeutic purpose this is called *essential oil synergy*. A synergistic essential oil blends total action is greater than any one of the essential oils independently.

Therapeutic blends a designed to help with a particular injury, illness, disease, a physical condition or an emotional condition. When the therapeutic value of the blend is the main focus, sometimes it's easy to not think about the aroma, but you can have both.

When you create a therapeutic blend, you need to consider all of the therapeutic values of a specific oil and make sure that you don't mix oils that will not work well together. For example, you have terrible muscle pain at night and it causes you trouble sleeping. You consider using peppermint with cypress, but both of these oils will energize you, even though they will help with your muscle pain.

It takes practice to get the art of blending essential oils perfected. You have to be not afraid to experiment and try. You are going to have some failures, but among those, you will also have some great hits.

As I mentioned earlier, there are different qualities of essential oils. Even when you are purchasing an essential oil marked therapeutic, there can still be significant differences. For example, lavender oil from different providers or different parts of the world can significantly vary in quality and effectiveness.

In addition to the therapeutic value of essential oils, they can be used in personal hygiene, beauty, insect repellents, diffusers, laundry cleaners, household products and more.

Blending Oils Based on Their Aroma

Essential oils can be categorized into broad groups based on their aromas. Here are some examples:

- **Earthy** – Patchouli, oak moss, vetiver
- **Floral** - Lavender, neroli, jasmine
- **Minty** – Spearmint, peppermint
- **Spicy** – Cinnamon, clove, nutmeg
- **Woodsy** – Cedar, pine
- **Herbaceous** – Basil, marjoram, rosemary
- **Oriental** – Patchouli, ginger
- **Citrus** – Lemon, orange, lime
- **Camphorous** – Tea tree, eucalyptus

Oils that are in the same aroma category will usually blend together well. However, there's no reason to just use oils together that are in the same broad category. Doing so would really constrict your creativity. To give you an idea of some of the things you might try:

1. Woodsy oils will blend nicely with every category.

2. Spicy oils will blend well with oriental, citrus and floral oils. Careful that you don't overpower the blend with spicy essential oils.

3. Oriental oils will blend well with spicy, citrus and floral oils. Careful that you don't overpower the blend with the oriental essential oils.

4. Florals will blend well with citrusy, woodsy and spicy essential oils.

5. Minty oils will blend well with citrus, earthy, woodsy and herbaceous essential oils.

Understanding Essential Oil Notes

An essential oil is assigned a note based on how fast it evaporates. An essential oil blend is placed on the skin can last differently. In some cases, it smells one way immediately, but completely different 4 hours later.

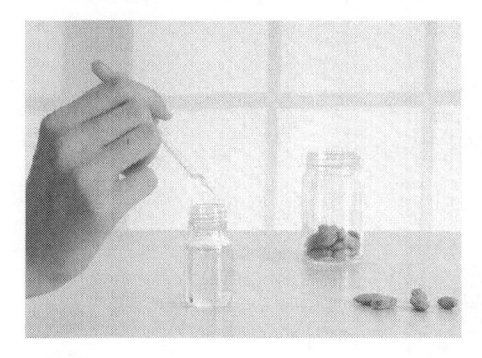

In other cases, within the hour there is no smell left at all. Fragrances smell different after time has passed. Essential oils have different evaporation rates. Top notes evaporate the fastest – generally within a couple of hours. Middle notes evaporate within 2 to 4 hours, while base notes last the longest.

Septimus Piesse actually created the odophone where odors were treated like sounds and a scale was created going from the lowest note to the highest note. If you find you have a true interest in getting the most out of blending essential oils, you may want to study this more. For now, let's look at some of the most common oils that fall into each category.

Top Notes

- Lavender
- Peppermint
- Lemon
- Bergamot
- Basil

- Eucalyptus
- Bay Laurel
- Citronella
- Spearmint
- Anise
- Orange
- Lemongrass
- Lime
- Grapefruit
- Tangerine

Middle Notes

- Ylang Ylang
- Jasmine
- Chamomile, Roman
- Chamomile, German
- Neroli
- Rose
- Geranium
- Hyssop
- Cinnamon
- Dill
- Fennel
- Tea Tree
- Clary Sage
- Nutmeg
- Clove Bud
- Cypress
- Marjoram
- Rosemary
- Parsley

- Juniper Berry
- Rose Geranium
- Scotch Pine
- Spruce
- Rosewood
- Yarrow
- Thyme
- Cajeput
- Black Pepper

Base Notes

- Frankincense
- Ginger
- Vanilla
- Myrrh
- Patchouli
- Sandalwood
- Cedarwood,
- Angelica Root
- Balsam, Peru
- Beeswax
- Olibanum
- Helichrysum (Immortelle)
- Benzoin
- Oak moss
- Vetiver

When you first begin to blend oils, starting with three essential oils is a great place to start. You choose a top note, middle note and base note. Then, as you gain experience, you can begin to increase the number of essential oils in your blends.

5 Things You Should Know About Blending Essential Oils

1. When you first begin to create your own blends, you should start by using only essential oils. You can add your carrier oil after you are happy with the blend you've created. In doing so you will not waste as much oil if you don't like something and it's much easier to keep adjusting when you are working with the pure oils.

2. When you first create a new blend of essential oils, begin with the smallest possible number of drops. Doing so not only wastes less oil it helps you to keep control on your mixture and tweak it the best.

3. Begin your blending trials, creating blends that are made up of essential oils where 20% are base notes, 30% are top notes, and 50% are middle notes.

4. Make sure that you always label your blends with exactly what's in them. If you do not have enough room on the bottle, then you need to keep a journal and use a numbering system so that you can always know what is in any blend and how many of each drop you added. You want to do this so you can later recreate something that works really well, change something that doesn't, and for any allergies or issues with essential oils, you need to know what's in a blend.

5. The best way to learn about an essential oil's strengths is by experimenting. Add one drop of your essential oil blend to 4 drops of carrier oil. This is a 20% dilution rate. Now you want to smell it, study the aroma and the therapeutic benefits.

   To obtain a 10% dilution rate, you just need to add 5 additional carrier oil drops. Then again, you will want to smell it, try it, experiment with it. This will help you learn the characteristics of your essential oil blend when it is diluted to different strengths.

How to Create Your Own First Aid Kit With Essential Oils

It's easy to put together a natural first aid kit using essential oils. You can easily treat the same things with your first aid kit built on essential oils, as you can with a typical first aid kit.

Essential oils are a much better choice, because they support your body and let it return to its natural state of balance. They are easy to use and you don't have to have a different first aid kit for the pets or children in your home. Everyone can use this.

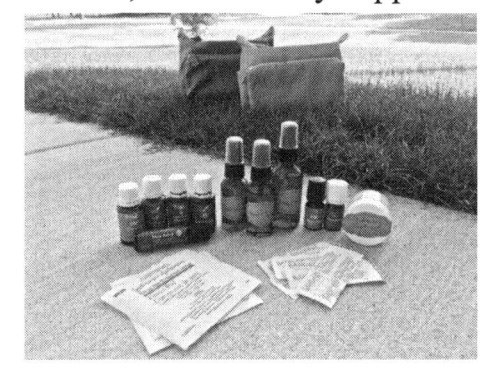

Each essential oil has a multiple of properties so it can be used to treat a number of conditions. This means with just 10-15 essential oils as your base, you'll be ready to treat most situations you'll run into.

Of course, in a real emergency, you need to call 911, and get medical help. However, even in these situations, there is a need for emotional support. You need to keep the injured party calm until help arrives and you can use essential oils to help achieve this.

Let's look at the main first aid situations you are likely to face and how you can treat them with essential oils.

Wound Healing With Essential Oils

Healing wounds naturally with essential oils is easy and it's highly effective. Use oils to treat, cuts, scrapes, puncture wounds, etc.

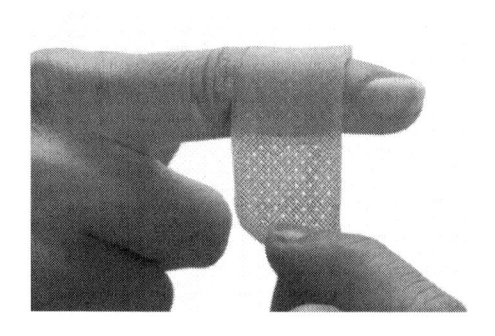

When you use commercial products to treat wounds, chemicals that do not belong in our body are absorbed and this actually can slow the healing process and create other situations like infection.

Many of these products are water based, and the skin repels water, so the product isn't properly absorbed into the skin to promote healing. Ointments and salves are usually petroleum based and that is not helpful for healing wounds. It actually clogs the skin and prevents penetration needed for healing.

Therapeutic grade essential oils help to speed up the healing process because of the combination of medicinal properties. Here are some of the properties you want when you are trying to heal wounds:

- Analgesic (pain relieving)
- Anti-bacterial
- Antibiotic
- Anti-fungal
- Anti-inflammatory

- Antiseptic
- Homeostatic (stops bleeding)
- Vulnerary (helps heal wounds)

All essential oils will have several of these properties, not just one. They have many benefits. Plus, you will be able to address trauma or shock.

Ingredients Found in Commercial Wound Ointments

Here are just a few ingredients that you will find in wound products. Most of these irritate the skin, are linked to allergies, suppress the immune system and some are even linked to cancer.

- Benzalkonium Chloride
- Butylated Hydroxytoluene (BHT)
- DMDM Hydantoin
- Mineral Oil
- Petrolatum
- Propylene Glycol
- Yellow #5; FD&C Blue #1

Sometimes commercially purchased products that claim to be natural will still contain some of these ingredients. Pet products are the worst, because they don't require any labeling.

The Best Essential Oils for Wound Healing

Select the essential oil you are going to use based on the type of wound and the action required.

To Disinfect:
- Tea Tree essential oil
- Thyme essential oil
- Oregano essential oil
- Hyssop essential oil

To Stop Bleeding:
- Helichrysum (The best to control bleeding) essential oil
- Geranium essential oil
- Rose Otto essential oil

To Treat Infected Wounds:
- Clove essential oil
- Myrrh essential oil

To Promote Healing:
- Tea Tree essential oil
- Lavender essential oil

To Help With Scarring:
- Lavender essential oil
- Geranium essential oil

Create a First Aid Spray:
- 10 drops lavender essential oil
- 6 drops tea tree essential oil
- 4 drops cypress essential oil

Instructions:
1. Place the essential oils in 1 teaspoon of salt.
2. Put 16 ounces of distilled water in a spray bottle.
3. Add the salt mixture.
4. Shake until dissolved.

Spray it on minor cuts, scrapes and wounds before you apply the bandages. You should spray throughout the day several times, for 4 days. You can also apply 1-2 drops of tea tree oil essential oil.

Treat Nausea and Vomiting With Essential Oils

Nausea and vomiting can be caused by a variety of digestive issues including parasites, constipation, food poisoning, motion sickness, indigestion or stomach flu.

There are different essential oils that can help depending on what the cause of your nausea or vomiting. If you are unsure of the cause, there are some general remedies that overlap. That's often a good place to start. However, if you know the cause, then it's better to choose an essential oil that's designed to work in that situation.

General Oils for Nausea and/or vomiting:
- Ginger essential oil
- Wintergreen essential oil
- Peppermint essential oil
- Nutmeg essential oil

Instructions:
Dilute and massage 2-3 drops behind the ear and around your navel area. Do this every hour. You can also use warm compresses over your stomach after you apply your essential oil. You can also inhale the oils as needed. Place 1 to 3 drops directly on your tongue and then swallow the water.

To Stop Vomiting:
- Patchouli essential oil – this is the best because it will

- Lavender essential oil
- Peppermint essential oil
- Nutmeg essential oil
- Fennel essential oil

Patchouli is one of the best oils for vomiting. It has highly effective compounds, because they decrease the gastrointestinal muscle contractions that are associated with vomiting.

Instructions:
Dilute and massage 2-3 drops behind the ear and around your navel area. Do this every hour. You can also use warm compresses over your stomach after you apply your essential oil. You can also inhale the oils as needed. Place 1 to 3 drops directly on your tongue and then swallow the water.

To Treat Morning Sickness and Motion Sickness
- Peppermint essential oil
- Ginger essential oil

Instructions:
Place 1-2 drops in a glass of water and sip slowly. You can also apply directly to your navel area. Dilute and massage 2-3 drops behind the ear and around your navel area. Do this every hour. You can also use warm compresses over your stomach after you apply your essential oil. You can also inhale the oils as needed. Place 1 to 3 drops directly on your tongue and then swallow the water.

To Treat Food Poisoning:

- Patchouli essential oil
- Peppermint essential oil
- Rosemary essential oil
- Tarragon essential oil

Instructions:

Place 1-2 drops in a glass of water and sip slowly. You can apply directly to your stomach area. Dilute and massage 2-3 drops behind the ear and around your stomach area. Do this every hour. You can also use warm compresses over your stomach after you apply your essential oil. You can inhale the oils as needed. Place 1 to 3 drops directly on your tongue and then swallow the water.

Reduce Jet Leg with Essential Oils

When you travel across time zones or body's circadian rhythms get all messed up. This can lead to insomnia, fatigue, headache and mental confusion.

These essential oils along with other techniques can help to reduce your jet lag.

- Geranium essential oil
- Lavender essential oil
- Eucalyptus essential oil
- Peppermint essential oil
- Clarity essential oil
- Grapefruit essential oil

Treating Minor Aches and Pain with Essential Oils

You exercise, you trip and twist something, you lift something too heavy – there are many reasons why you find yourself dealing with minor aches and pain. Essential oils can help.

Chronic pain, as a result of autoimmune disorders like fibromyalgia or degenerative disorders like arthritis, the relief are more difficult to treat and a combination of essential oils with other natural treatments will give you the best results.

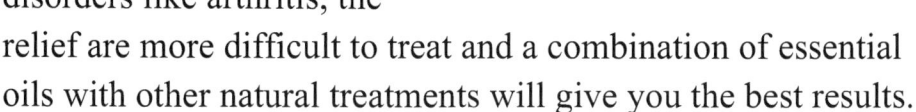

- Wintergreen essential oil
- Helichrysum essential oil
- Clover essential oil
- Peppermint essential oil
- Pine essential oil
- Lavender essential oil
- Ginger essential oil
- Cinnamon essential oil

Instructions:

If you make a blend of wintergreen, helichrysum, clover and peppermint you will get maximum benefits. Lavender disinfects and can also help a wound start to heal quickly along with relieving pain.

Ease Muscle Spasms with Essential Oils

Essential oils work best to prevent injury or muscle spasms, but if you find yourself dealing with muscle spasms, there are some excellent essential oils that work as a muscle relaxer.

- Marjoram essential oil
- Basil essential oil
- Roman Chamomile essential oil
- Wintergreen essential oil
- Helichrysum essential oil
- Clover essential oil
- Peppermint essential oil

Instructions:
Again, making a blend from the last four give excellent results. Mix your essential oils 50:50 with your carrier oil. Apply at least three times a day. You can also alternate between hot and cold packs to increase the relief from strained muscles. Light stretching can also be beneficial.

Essential Oils That Have a Cooling Effect:
- Eucalyptus essential oil
- Peppermint essential oil
- Wintergreen essential oil

Essential Oils That Have a Warming Effect:
- Thyme essential oil

- Marjoram essential oil
- Basil essential oil
- Helichrysum essential oil
- Roman Chamomile essential oil
- Clove essential oil
- Black Pepper essential oil
- Capsicum essential oil

Treat Bee Stings and Bites with Essential Oils

You can quickly and easily address bee stings with essential oils. Essential oils have antihistamine and anti-inflammatory properties that are excellent for dealing with bee or wasp stings. Of course, if you are allergic to bees then you need to seek immediate medical help.

To Treat Bee or Wasp Stings:

- Roman chamomile essential oil
- Lavender essential oil
- Peppermint essential oil
- Tea tree essential oil

Wasps and hornets don't leave their stinger. However, bees do, so if a bee has stung you, first you will need to remove the stinger, and then apply 1-2 drops to the bite. For the first hour apply every 15 minutes and then apply 3-4 times a day until swelling and redness is gone. You can also apply a cold compress.

Because of the alkaline nature of wasp venom, a blend of 3 drops lavender essential oil, 3 drops Roman chamomile essential oil and 2 drops basil essential oil with 1 teaspoon of apple cider vinegar is generally more effective.

To Treat Mosquito Bites Use:
- Lavender essential oil
- Helichrysum essential oil

Another recipe for bites and stings is this poultice:
- 18 drops lavender essential oil
- 7 drops chamomile essential oil
- 1 ½ tablespoon bentonite clay
- 1 ½ teaspoon tincture
- 3 teaspoons distilled water

Instructions:
Mix and blend and then apply the paste to the bite. It helps to remove toxins and provides relief from itching and pain.

Treat Minor Burns with Essential Oils

You can easily treat minor burns at home. However, if you have suffered a major burn, you need to see a doctor immediately. Essential oils do an excellent job of soothing minor burns.

To Treat Minor Burns Use:
- Helichrysum essential oil
- Lavender essential oil
- Rose essential oil
- Frankincense essential oil
- Aloe vera essential oil

Instructions:
Lavender and aloe vera can be applied directly to the burn without reducing with a carrier oil.

Treat Sunburn with Essential Oils

Sunburn is never fun, in fact, it can be quite painful. The sooner you address it the better.

To Treat Sunburn:
- Lavender essential oil
- Helichrysum essential oil
- Tea tree essential oil
- Rose essential oil

These four essential oils make an excellent blend for treating sunburn. There is no question that lavender is the best oil for sunburn relief. It's also important that you draw the heat out of your body. You can do that by making a mixture of:

- 2 cups apple cider vinegar (or white vinegar will work)
- Ice cubes
- 10 drops of lavender essential oil

Instructions:
1. Fill a bath or sink with tepid water.
2. Add the 2 cups of apple cider vinegar.
3. Immerse yourself for 20-30 minutes or as long as you can tolerate.
4. Once you are in the bath, if you can tolerate the temperature, add the ice cubes to your water.
5. Gently pat dry.
6. Now apply undiluted Lavender essential over the burned area. You can also use aloe vera in areas that burned the worst.

Treating Sunburn in Children

If you are treating sunburn in children you can use the recipe above. But you also want to keep your child cool and dry to try to prevent heat rash. Clothing made from light, natural fabrics is best. Expose as much skin as possible to air. If your child does develop heat rash.

Heat Rash Relief

Children Ages 0-4
- ½ cup baking soda
- 4 drops Lavender essential oil

Children Ages 5–10
- 1 cup baking soda
- 8 drops Lavender essential oil

Children Ages 11–18
- 2 cups baking soda
- 8 drops Lavender essential oil

Instructions:
1. Mix the lavender essential oil with the baking soda.
2. Add the mixture to a warm bath.
3. If you are bathing a baby, check to see that the folds of the skin have contact with the water.
4. Gently pat dry.

Warnings:
- When you are applying lavender essential oil to the burn, apply just a light layer, do not over apply.
- Do not use soap or bubble bath as this will dry your skin out and irritate it.
- Try to avoid anything that will irritate your sunburn such as rubbing to dry off.

Calming With Essential Oils

After an accident or injury a person can become very distressed, worried, agitated and anxious. You can use essential oils to calm them while you treat them or while you wait for help to arrive.

- Lavender
- Roman chamomile
- Patchouli
- Orange
- Ylang ylang
- Tangerine
- Cedarwood

All of these can work when you need to calm someone, so grab what you have handy. You can either use the tissue method (discussed earlier), where you put a couple of drops on a tissue and they inhale, or you can put a couple of drop on their neck, wrist, and/or temples.

Wrapping it All Up

I have given you the basics to create your own first aid kit including essential oil. I have given you some guidance on how to use the essential oils and treat the situation at hand.

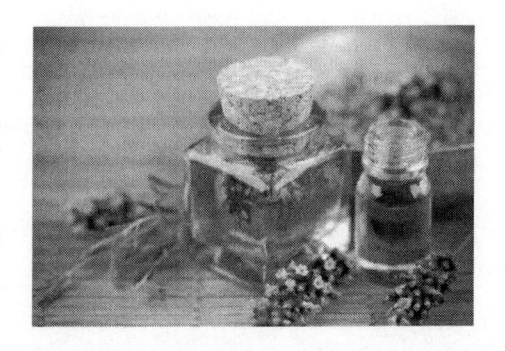

However, it is important to remember that this is not a first aid course. I encourage everyone to take a basic first aid course, so that in the case of an emergency, you are equipped to handle the situation at hand.

You do, however, have enough information here to handle the bumps and bruises that are part of everyday life for you and your family.

Calming Emotions Using Essential Oils

Many of us are not aware of just how powerful scent is and how it affects us. You have five senses and your sense of smell is the only one that is connected to the limbic system of the brain, which is your emotional control center. This is why scent can impact your emotions and how your body responds physically. Mood is important.

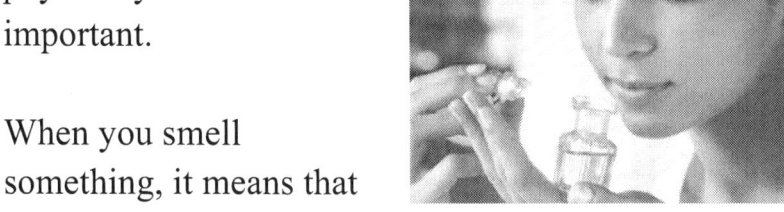

When you smell something, it means that miniscule molecules have evaporated from something and have entered your nose. Essential oils are volatile, which means they will evaporate at room temperature; so it means that these tiny little molecules literally jump through the air. When you inhale a smell, it channels these molecules through your nostrils, which sends a message to the receptors of your olfactory system. In turn you 'smell.' The same applies with essential oils.

Have you ever walked into a place, smelled something and instantly had a flashback to something in your childhood? Maybe you think of your home or your grandma's house? Perhaps you walk past someone and the perfume they are wearing reminds you of someone? Scent is powerful.

The limbic system is connected to the area of your brain responsible for blood pressure, heart rate, stress levels, digestion, breathing, hormone balance and sexual arousal. So, it makes sense that the use of therapeutic essential oils in aromatherapy could have significant psychological and physiological effects on both our physical and our emotional well-being, healing to our mind, body and soul.

Did you know that when you are stressed the physical response you have, can actually be measured. Stress and anxiety can affect your skin, lower your energy, affect your digestion, irritate your nerves and muscles, interfere with sleep and make you more likely to get sick.

Therapeutic essential oils are a safe and effective way to help to reset your emotions so that they are balanced, without the side effects many prescription drugs have.

Let's look at essential oils that affect the emotions and what their strong points are.

1. **Valerian** – Calms and can help with sleep.
2. **Frankincense** – Encourages feelings of joy and happiness.
3. **Bergamot** – Relieves anxiety, agitation and sadness.
4. **Neroli** – A relaxant that can calm, help you cope, and lift your spirits. It can also help with exaggerated or uncontrolled emotions, sadness and occasional sleeplessness. A natural relaxant used to help calm, uplift and it will also help you to cope with negative emotions.

5. **Vetiver** – It can help with occasional anxiety, sadness, stress and it can help you to recover from an upsetting occurrence or event.
6. **Lemon and Orange** – Helps to normalize stress.
7. **Tangerine** – Calming and sedating, so works well for anxiety and nervous feelings.

In addition to using essential oils, you should:

- Make sure you are drinking plenty of water.
- Get enough sleep.
- Drink plenty of water.
- Eat a well-balanced diet
- Pray or meditate.
- Stay away from processed foods, dyes, sugars, etc.
- Take your multivitamin.
- Detoxify your home.
- Make sure you are getting enough of the B vitamins and vitamin D.
- Learn relaxation techniques.

Next, I are going to begin to build a recipe section, so that by the time you are done reading this book, you can make the products you use in your home. Not only will you save tons of money, you will be using products that are healthy and effective. Are you ready? Great, let's move on.

40 Aromatherapy Recipes You Can Make at Home

1. Bath Salts Recipe

Many of us like our baths! They are relaxing and can even be invigorating. What could be better that some bath salts to help eliminate the days aches and pains.

What You Need:
3 cups salt Himalayan pink salt, sea salt, epsom salt or dead sea salt. You can use one or combine as many as you like.

Salts come in different sizes. The larger the salts the longer it takes for them to dissolve. Mid to small grain sizes work best.

If you are using larger pieces rather than measuring out, you can put larger pieces in your bath and then remove what has not dissolved. However, this is a much less economical way of doing it.

Then you want to add 20 drops of your favorite essential oil or essential oil blend.

If you want to moisturize just add 3 tablespoons of coconut oil.

Directions:

1. Take the salt and put it into a glass bowl.
2. Add your essential oil and use a fork to make sure it's mixed well.
3. If you are going to add coconut oil, add it now too.
4. You can actually store your salts; just put a lid on that seals tight.
5. Begin to fill your bath and when there is about 3" of water, you can pour 1 cup of salts into the tub. Swirl the water to make sure they mix well.
6. Jump in and enjoy!

2. Homemade Lotion Recipe

Most of us, at least women, like to put on a nice light moisturizer to help keep our skin soft and supple, and to keep those wrinkles at bay.

The trouble is most of the products you buy at the store are going to be filled with chemicals and preservatives.

This great little recipe can be used on your face and body. It contains no chemicals and it's ability to penetrate deep into the skin is extremely beneficial.

What You Need:
- Glass jars with lids that seal
- Double boiler
- Saucepan
- Whisk

Ingredients:
- ½ cup of carrier oil
- 3 teaspoons Vitamin E
- 4 tablespoons emulsifying wax depending on how thick you want it
- ½ -cup distilled water
- ½ teaspoon stearic acid
- 30 drops of your favorite essential oil

- 15 drops grapefruit seed extract as a natural preservative

Directions:
1. Add the oil, emulsifying wax and stearic acid together in the top of your double boiler
2. Put on low heat and warm slowly. You will need to keep stirring it until the way is all melted.
3. Remove from the heat and add the Vitamin E.
4. Take your saucepan and pour the water into it.
5. Heat on medium until it's lukewarm.
6. Slowly pour the water into the oil while stirring briskly using your whisk until it is a uniform color.
7. Now add your essential oils and the grapefruit seed extract.
8. Keep mixing.
9. When you are sure it is well mixed you can pour your body lotion into your glass bottles.
10. While its cooling, the oil and water are going to separate. You will need to shake the mixture every 5-6 minutes to make sure that it stays mixed – This is a very IMPORTANT step. After the lotion is completely cooled, it will no longer separate.
11. Store in a dark, cool place.

3. Massage Oil Recipe – 4 Options

Massage oils are an excellent way to deliver therapeutic benefits from the essential oils and, in addition, massage can relax and distress the body.

Massages can also be a sensual experience and are a great way for a couple to build intimacy. There are many different blends that can be used in massage. The four I have provided are just the beginning. If you, or you and your partner, have a favorite essential oil, make up your own massage oil blend.

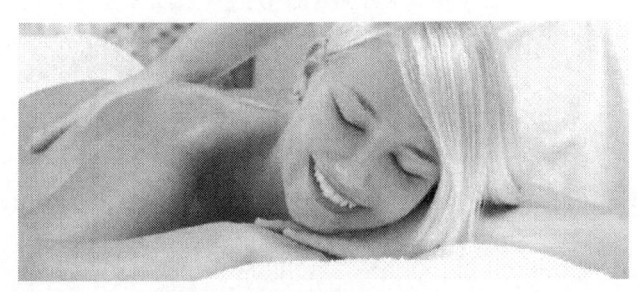

What You Need:
- Glass bowl
- Glass jars or bottles that seal

Ingredients:
- 3 ounces of Sweet Almond Oil
- 45-50 drops of essential oils. (see below)

1. **Sleep Blend** - 45 drops Roman chamomile.
2. **Stress Blend** – 36 drops lavender, 4 drops lemon, 10 drops clary sage.
3. **Sore Muscle Blend** - 15 drops peppermint, 15 drops eucalyptus, 5 drops black pepper, 5 drops ginger.

4. **Aphrodisiac Blend** – 30 drops sandalwood, 10 drops jasmine.

Directions:
1. Mix your oils and essential oils together well.
2. Pour into your glass jars or bottles and seal.
3. Store in a dark place.

Place a small amount of oil in your hand and begin the massage. I have assumed that you already know the correct techniques for massage. If you do not, please learn those first.

4. Aromatherapy Bath Oil Recipe

You might be tempted to just the essential oils right into your bath water, but the trouble is they won't disperse evenly and you risk a concentrated amount landing on your skin. This recipe for a bath oil, is simple to make and store. It moisturizes your skin as you bath.

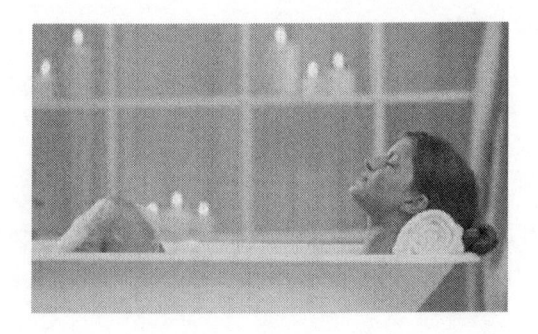

The majority of bath oil products you buy contain synthetic ingredients to help disperse the oils into the water so that they are mixed. This recipe contains no additives, and does not use a chemical dispersing agent.

What You Need:
- Glass bottles that seal.
- Large glass measuring cup

Ingredients:
- 8 fl. ounces carrier oil such as jojoba
- 100 drops of lavender essential oil

Directions:
1. Blend the oils together in a large glass measuring cup.
2. Pour into glass bottles and seal.

Run your bathwater, and once there is about 3" of water in your bath, you can add about ¼ ounce of your bath oil, then swirl with your hand to ensure it is evenly mixed through the water. Relax and enjoy!

Using this bath oil blend is safer than just adding pure essential oils directly to the bath water. It reduces the potential of the undiluted essential oils settling in one spot on your skin and causing an irritation.

5. Peppermint Rosemary Shampoo

The commercial blends of shampoo you buy are filled with chemicals that are toxic. Sodium lauryl sulfate, which is a known carcinogen, is what makes commercial shampoos lather.

This is a great alternative. Your hair will be squeaky clean and you'll eliminate the health risks. You will also save a ton of money, because this shampoo is cheap to make.

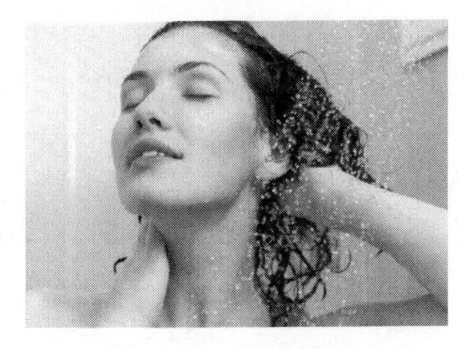

What You Need:
- Container with a flip top – an old rinsed shampoo bottle will work.

Ingredients:
- 2 cups castile soap
- 2 cups distilled or filtered water
- 50 drops rosemary essential oil
- 20 drops peppermint essential oil

Instructions:
1. Add the castile soap to your container.
2. Add the Rosemary and Peppermint essential oils.
3. Add the water and gently turn to mix.

Shampoo and rinse as normal.

6. Hair Conditioner

You Will Need:
- Glass bowl to mix or large measuring cup
- Funnel
- Glass bottles that seal

Ingredients:
- 3 cups jojoba
- 75 drops rosemary essential oil

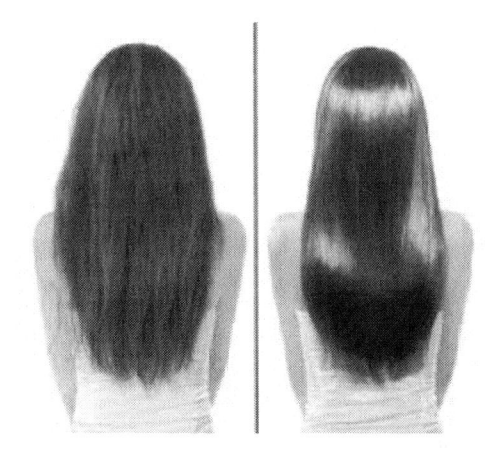

Directions:
1. The recipe makes one dose. You can increase and store in a glass bottle if you'd like to keep on hand.
2. Mix the Jojoba and rosemary essential oil in a small bowl.
3. Wet your hair with warm water and then apply the conditioning blend. Leave on your hair for 30-45 minutes. Then, wash your hair as normal.

Jojoba and rosemary benefit dry hair. Rosemary essential oil is also helpful in dandruff.

Rather than just making a single usage, you can multiply the recipe and make yourself a full bottle of hair conditioner so you have it handy any time you wash your hair.

7. Acne Recipe

The commercial acne products on the market are harsh and contain all kinds of chemicals. Why not try a natural, safe and effective alternative.

What You Need;
- Glass measuring cup
- Glass bottles that seal

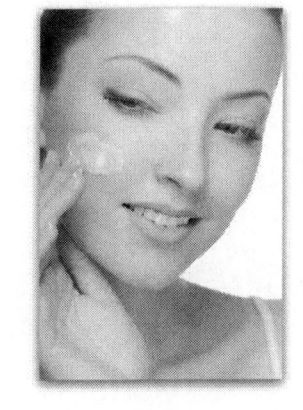

Ingredients:
- 4 fl. ounce jojoba
- 32 drops lavender essential oil
- 20 drops tea tree essential oil

Directions:
1. Pour the jojoba and essential oils into the glass measuring cup. Stir well.
2. Pour into your glass bottles and place the lid on tightly.
3. Gently roll the bottle back & forth for 1-2 minutes to mix the oils.

Gently roll the bottle before to each use. Dab a small amount onto areas of acne.

8. Sugar Facial and Body Scrub

Natural sugar scrubs are a great option for exfoliating. They are less abrasive than commercial scrubs and they have no chemicals. They will gently polish and exfoliate your skin. They are luxurious and smell delicious.

Over time, the ingredients tend to separate and they can also quickly harbor bacteria.

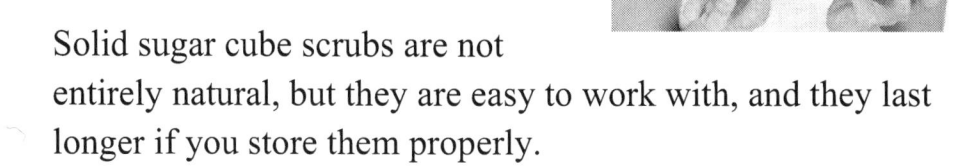

Solid sugar cube scrubs are not entirely natural, but they are easy to work with, and they last longer if you store them properly.

What You Need:
- Double boiler
- Glass mixing bowl
- Soap molds

Ingredients:
- 12 oz. Melt & Pour Soap Base
- 3 cups white sugar
- 20-25 drops of your favorite essential oil
- 3 fl. oz. coconut oil
- ½ tsp. Vitamin E oil

Directions:

1. Measure your ingredients out. You need to have them ready for when the soap is melted.
2. Place your Melt & Pour Soap Base in the top of your double boiler and on low-med heat gently melt it, until it is completely melted. DO NOT overheat it, as it will ruin your lather.
3. Immediately when it is melted, pour it into your mixing bowl.
4. Now add other ingredients you prepared.
5. As you add the sugar, you need to be constantly stirring.
6. If the mixture isn't thick enough, add more sugar. It might take some trial and error to get the consistency you like.
7. Spoon the mixture into the soap molds. Press so that all the air pockets are removed.
8. Let stand 1-2 hours.
9. Once they are firmed up, they will release from the molds.
10. Cut into 1" cubes.
11. Let firm up at room temperature overnight.

9. Cuticle Oil

Here's the perfect way to keep your cuticles soft and healthy. Most commercial products contain alcohol. Unless you make it yourself, it's hard to find a product that's all oil.

What You Need:
- 2 – 2 ounce glass jars with lids.
- Glass measuring cup

Ingredients:
- 4 ounces cold pressed carrier oil.
- 40-50 drops of either lavender or sandalwood essential oil.

Directions:
1. Add your carrier oil and essential oils together in a measuring cup.
2. Mix well.
3. Pour into your glass jars.
4. Mix before each use by gently turning.

Brush onto your cuticles the skin around your cuticles. Massage in. Apply 1-2 times a week. Since there are no preservatives, the shelf life is about a month. You can decrease the recipe size if you like.

10. Rose Oil Aphrodisiac

The rose essential oil is intoxicating, which makes this a terrific aphrodisiac. It works well to relieve stress.

Ingredients:
- 6 drops of rose essential oil
- 3 drops of sandalwood
- 8 tablespoons heavy cream

Directions:
For a relaxing bath, mix your essential oils and heavy cream together in measuring cup or small bowl and then add it directly to your bath.

Aromatherapy Perfume Recipes

When you blend essential oils to create a fragrance that you like, it allows you to mix creativity and science. You get to enjoy the fragrance and the therapeutic benefits. However, for perfumes the focus is on the final fragrance, not the therapeutic properties.

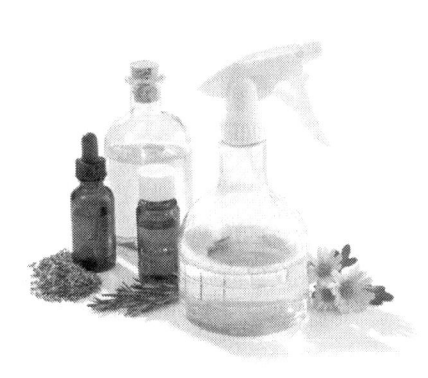

Remember to always follow safety precautions when you are blending. For example, if you created a fragrance with bergamot you would need to be careful as it has significant phototoxic properties. In other words, you need to know your oils.

Traditional perfumers who work at worldly fragrance houses have studied for years to master their art and they are the rare group that really understands perfumery science.

Perfumers understand both essential oils and synthesized chemicals, which are used to mimic the chemicals of essential oils because they are much cheaper than pure essential oils and also because they can be standardized so that they consistently get an identical aroma.

In aromatherapy, only natural ingredients are blended to create a perfume.

11. Perfume Recipe

Ingredients:
- 1 drop of jasmine
- 7 drops sandalwood
- 1 tablespoon jojoba

Directions:
1. Blend the oils together.
2. Store in a dark-colored glass container and seal.

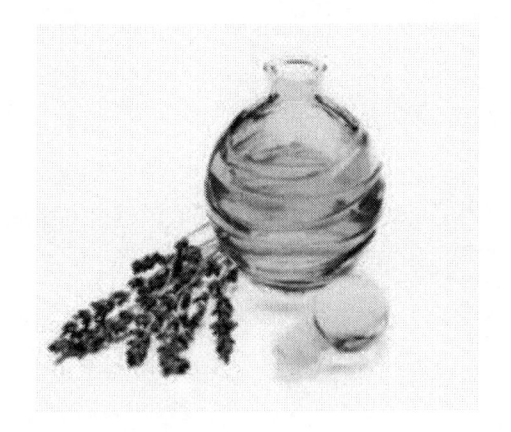

Dab a drop onto your pulse area.

12. Alcohol or Water Base Perfume Recipe

What You Need:
- Dark-colored glass container.
- Coffee filter
- Small glass bottles with eye droppers

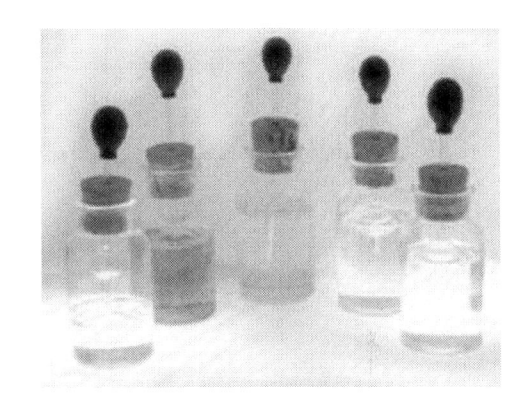

Ingredients:
- 10 teaspoons vodka
- 5 teaspoons distilled water
- 40-60 drops of your perfume blend

Directions:
1. Blend all your ingredients together and mix well.
2. Store in an airtight dark-colored glass container.
3. Let sit for 3 weeks and each day shake the mixture 4-5 times. The more you shake it the better your perfumes going to be.
4. At the end of the 3 weeks, you can use a coffee filter to filter your perfume through and rebottle it.

You are only going to need a really, small amount of this as it has a heavy concentration of essential oils.

13. Carrier Oil Base Perfume Recipe

Ingredients:
- 16-20 drops of your perfume blend
- 2 tablespoons jojoba

Directions:
1. Blend your ingredients together.
2. Store in a sealed dark-colored bottle.
3. Dab a drop onto your pulse points.

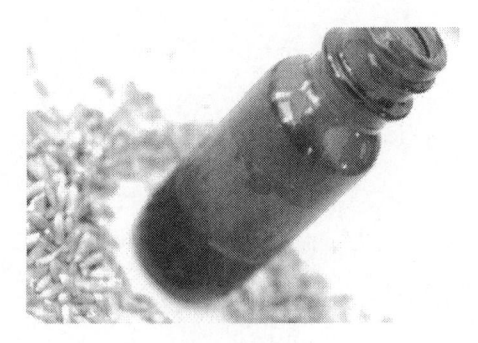

This blend has a heavy concentration of essential oils so use it sparingly. Always check the safety data for the oils in your blend and do a skin test before you use it.

14. Cologne Recipe

Ingredients:
- 5 teaspoons vodka
- 25-35 drops of your perfume blend
- 3 teaspoons distilled water

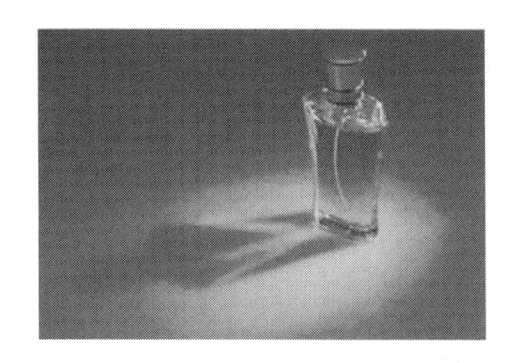

Directions:
1. Blend all your ingredients together and make sure you mix them really good.
2. Store in a sealed dark-colored glass container.
3. Let sit for 3 weeks and each day shake the mixture 4-5 times. The more you shake it the better your perfumes going to be.
4. At the end of the 3 weeks, you can use a coffee filter to filter your perfume through and rebottle it.

This blend has a heavy concentration of essential oils so use it sparingly.

15. Body Splash Recipe

Ingredients:
- 10 teaspoons Vodka
- 5 teaspoons Distilled Water
- 18-30 drops of your perfume blend

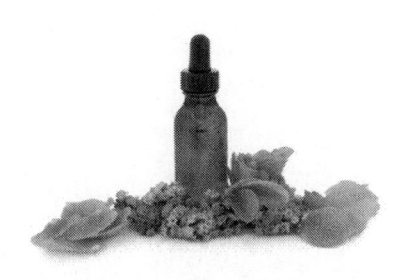

Directions:
1. Mix all the ingredients together and make sure they are well blended.
2. Store in a sealed dark-colored glass container.
3. Let sit for 3 weeks and each day shake the mixture 4-5 times. The more you shake it the better your perfumes going to be.
4. At the end of the 3 weeks, you can use a coffee filter to filter your perfume through and rebottle it.

Aromatherapy Recipes for Around Your House

Your home is a where you spend a great deal of your time with friends and family. It's where you create memories. If you are reading this book, it's evident you are looking to create a healthier lifestyle that promotes wellness for you and your family and part of that is creating a safe, healthy, calm and relaxing home environment to live in.

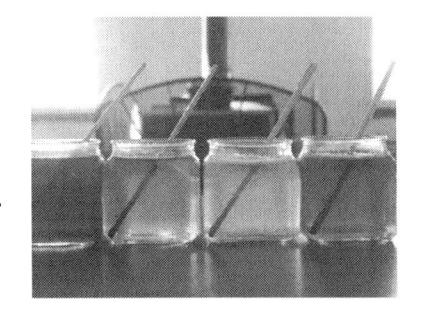

Essential oils are a great alternative to products containing synthetic ingredients and toxic chemicals. Let's get started with some recipes for around the home.

16. Aromatherapy Room Mister Air Fresheners

Here are a few easy-to-make room mists and air freshener recipes.

You can always make up your own blends, or you can use a single essential oil, but this will get you started. Even though you are making air fresheners, you should still make sure you are using therapeutic quality oils.

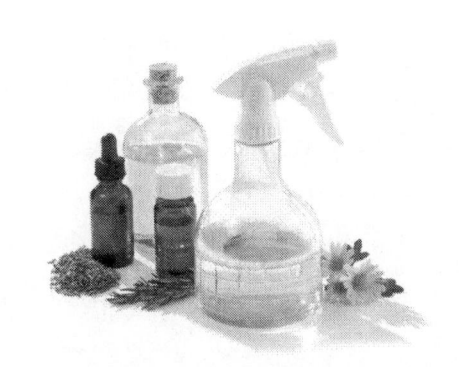

1. Take an 8 oz. clean glass spray bottle that has a mister. You want to use glass because the essential oils can pull toxins out of the plastic. You will add only 6 oz of liquids so that there is room to shake well.
2. Take 40-70 drops of your favorite essential oil or essential oil blend. Essential oils can vary in strength. You might want to start with the lowest number of drops and then keep adding drops until you find the right aroma for you and your family, especially if you are sensitive to strong aromas.
3. Add 3 ounces of distilled water and 3 ounces of high-proof alcohol. You can leave out the alcohol and increase the amount of distilled water to 6 ounces, but it is the alcohol that helps keep the aroma lingering in the air for longer. You can use vodka or everclear as your alcohol, but never use rubbing alcohol because it almost always will contain additives that will contaminate your blend.

4. Shake the bottle before you use it and lightly mist your room.
5. Try it for the first time, but wait a day or two before you decide if the aroma is right. Aromas change with time.

Blend #1
- 4 drops peppermint
- 8 drops spearmint
- 12 drops grapefruit
- 22 drops rosemary

Blend #2
- 15 drops lemon
- 12 drops lavender
- 10 drops clary sage

Blend #3
- 30 drops lime
- 12 drops ylang ylang
- 6 drops bergamot
- 6 drops rose

Blend #3
- 25 drops spearmint
- 20 drops bergamot

17. Aromatherapy Essential Oil Diffuser Blends – Mood Setters

First, create the diffuser blend by adding the appropriate amount of essential oil(s) to a dark-colored glass bottle. Then follow the manufactures instructions on the diffuser and add the required number of blended drops to your diffuser.

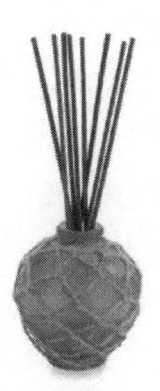

Before you use thicker essential oils like patchouli or sandalwood, in your nebulizing diffuser, I suggest that you carefully read your diffuser's instructions.

The goal of these diffuser recipes is to appeal to your senses and create a positive mood. These blends are not designed to be therapeutic, just smell nice.

Blend #1
- 3 drops cinnamon
- 3 drops jasmine
- 2 drops sweet orange
- 2 drops lime

Blend #2
- 8 drops of patchouli
- 5 drops of vanilla

- 1 drop of neroli

Blend #3
- 10 drops lime
- 6 drops bergamot
- 3 drops rose
- 3 drops ylang ylang

Blend #4
- 10 drops lavender
- 6 drops bergamot
- 2 drops cypress

Blend #5
- 5 drops ylang ylang
- 4 drops bergamot
- 1 drop grapefruit
- 1 drop lemon

Blend #6
- 4 drops lavender
- 3 drops rosemary
- 2 drops peppermint
- 1 drop roman chamomile

Blend #7
- 7 drops sandalwood
- 4 drops bergamot
- 3 drops jasmine
- 1 drop grapefruit

Blend #8
- 8 drops lavender
- 3 drops ylang ylang
- 1 drop rosewood

Blend #9
- 8 drops spruce
- 3 drops lavender
- 3 drops cedar

Blend #10
- 14 drops lemon
- 8 drops bergamot
- 2 drops spearmint

Blend #11
- 7 drops juniper
- 3 drops cinnamon
- 2 drops sweet orange

Blend #12
- 12 drops sweet orange
- 4 drops spearmint
- 2 drops lavender

Blend #13
- 8 drops sandalwood
- 2 drops scotch pine
- 1 drop rose

- 1 drop lemon

Blend #15
- 10 drops sweet orange
- 4 drops vanilla
- 1 drop ylang ylang

Blend #16
- 7 drops sandalwood
- 2 drops scotch pine
- 1 drop rose
- 1 drop lemon

18. Aromatherapy Essential Oil Diffuser Blends – Therapeutic

First, create the diffuser blend by adding the appropriate amount of essential oil(s) to a dark-colored glass bottle. Then follow the manufactures instructions on the diffuser and add the required number of blended drops to your diffuser.

Before you use thicker essential oils like patchouli or sandalwood, in your nebulizing diffuser, it's a good idea for you to carefully read your diffuser's instructions.

The goal of these diffuser recipes is to appeal to your senses and create a positive mood. These blends are designed to have therapeutic value, unlike the previous group.

Blend #1 For Chest and Sinus Congestion
- 4 drops eucalyptus
- 3 drops tea tree
- 2 drops lavender

Blend #2 For Colds
- 4 drops eucalyptus
- 3 drops rosemary
- 2 drops lavender

Blend #3 Sinus Congestion
- 4 drops Eucalyptus
- 3 drops peppermint
- 2 drops tea tree

Blend #4 Coughs
- 4 drops eucalyptus
- 4 drops lavender

Blend #5 Headache
- 10 drops lavender
- 4 drops chamomile
- 2 drops peppermint

Blend #6 Eliminate Allergies
- 4 drops peppermint
- 4 drops lavender
- 4 drops lemon

Blend #7 Reduce Stress
- 8 drops lavender
- 6 drops clary sage
- 2 drops marjoram
- 2 drops ylang ylang

19. Aromatherapy Essential Oil Diffusion for Gratitude

Combine the essential oils in a clean glass bottle and then diffuse as you normally would. Feel free to experiment with the blend.

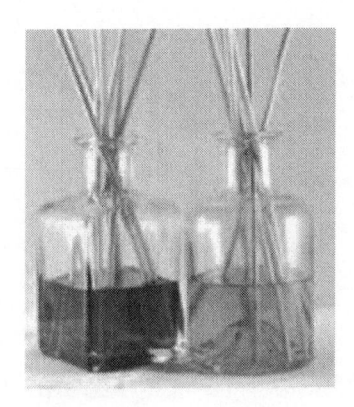

Recipe
- 20 drops bergamot – enhances joy
- 18 drop frankincense – creates balance
- 10 drops ylang ylang – exotic floral
- 8 drops cypress - energizing
- 8 drops grapefruit - uplifting
- 3 drops ginger – uplifting
- 4 drops jasmine – exotic floral

Recipes for Therapeutic Aromatherapy

Therapeutic aromatherapy is a huge part of aromatherapy. In essence using essential oils through aromatherapy allows the creation of many natural medicines.

There are so many different blends that can be created to deal with physical ailments, illness, injury and emotional troubles.

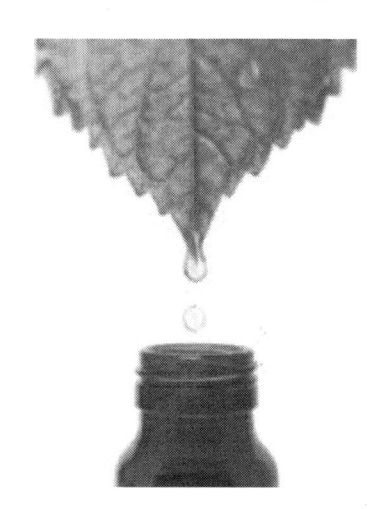

I am going to provide you with numerous recipes that you can use on yourself and your family.

Preparing Your Essential Oils

Earlier we looked at different ways to use aromatherapy. **Most essential oils should not be applied to your skin directly in their pure form.** In the majority of cases, you will dilute with a carrier oil or sometimes with water, so that the concentration is between 3% and 5%.

For example, if you have one teaspoon of carrier oil, you would add between 3 and 5 drops of your essential oil. If you are using water as your carrier, you will need to shake every time before applying, as it separates from the oil.

You should always review any safety data on essential oils and essential oil blends, especially if you are taking any other medications, prescription or over the counter.

5 Application Methods

1. Compress
Dilute your essential oil(s) with your carrier oil or water. Then apply to the affected area. You can also apply to a dressing before applying to the area. The compress can be applied hot or cold.

2. Bath
You can add your essential oil(s) directly to your bath water according to the recipe you have used. You will add the oils just prior to getting into the bath. This manner allows the essential oils to be absorbed throughout your skin and you will get the additional benefit of inhaling the essential oil(s).

3. Gargle
Add a few drops of your essential oil to water. Stir and gargle like normal. Do not swallow the mixture. Begin with one drop and you can increase from there. That way you'll be able to find the right strength so it is not too strong.

4. Diffuser Blends

Multiply your blend by 4x to obtain the strength that it should be to use in a diffuser. Always follow the manufacturer's instructions.

5. **Massage**

For massage to apply to bigger areas of the body, a 1% solution is adequate. This means 1 teaspoon of oil would get 1 drop of essential oil.

Use one of these methods for the therapeutic blends that follow.

20. Recipes to Relieve Anger

These blends can help when you are angry.

Blend #1
- 6 drops bergamot
- 3 drops ylang ylang
- 3 drops jasmine

Blend #2
- 3 drops rose
- 2 drops orange
- 2 drops vetiver

Blend #3
- 4 drops patchouli
- 3 drops orange

Blend #4
- 5 drops orange
- 3 drops bergamot
- 2 drops Roman chamomile

21. Recipes to Calm Anxiety

These blends will help if you are dealing with anxiety.

Blend #1
- 5 drops lavender
- 3 drops clary sage

Blend #2
- 4 drops bergamot
- 3 drops frankincense
- 2 drops clary sage

Blend #3
- 4 drops lavender
- 2 drops mandarin
- 2 drops rose
- 2 drops vetiver

Blend #4
- 6 drops bergamot
- 2 drops sandalwood

22. Recipes to Increase Confidence

These blends will help you increase your confidence.

Blend #1
- 3 drops cypress
- 2 drops grapefruit

Blend #2
- 4 drops rosemary
- 2 drops orange

Blend #3
- 8 drops bergamot
- 6 drops jasmine

Blend #4
- 5 drops bergamot
- 2 drops bay laurel

23. Recipes to Calm and Relax

These blends will help you to calm and relax.

Blend #1
- 4 drops frankincense
- 2 drops Roman chamomile
- 3 drops lavender

Blend #2
- 12 drops Roman chamomile
- 3 drops lavender

24. Recipes to Ease Depression

These blends will help during times of depression.

Blend #1
- 6 drops sandalwood
- 2 drops orange
- 2 drops rose

Blend #2
- 5 drops bergamot
- 2 drops clary sage

Blend #3
- 4 drops frankincense
- 2 drop lemon
- 2 drops jasmine
- 1 drops neroli

Blend #4
- 4 drops ylang ylang
- 2 drops lavender
- 1 drops grapefruit

25. Recipes to Increase Energy

These blends will help to increase your energy.

Blend #1
5 drops rosemary
3 drops bergamot

Blend #2
3 drops frankincense
2 drops lemon
1 drop peppermint

Blend #3
5 drops ginger
1 drop grapefruit

Blend #4
3 drops cypress
2 drops grapefruit
2 drops basil

26. Recipe to Reduce Menstrual Cramps

If you are dealing with menstrual cramps, several essential oils that can help. Don't be afraid to experiment. Add a few drops to a warm bath with a some epsom salt, or add a few drops to a carrier oil and rub directly throughout your abdominal area.

Essential oils that are useful for menstrual cramps:

- Lavender
- Chamomile
- Frankincense
- Peppermint
- Jasmine
- Rosemary
- Clary Sage
- Basil
- Cypress
- Juniper
- Marjoram
- Nutmeg

27. Recipe to Reduce the Symptoms For Cold & Flu

What You Need:
- Large bowl
- Towel

Ingredients:
- 10 drops eucalyptus essential oil
- 6 drops scotch pine essential oil
- 6 drops lemon essential oil
- Boiling water

Instructions:
1. Boil your water and pour into a large bowl.
2. Add all the essential oils to the steaming water.
3. Covering your head with a towel and lean over the bowl. Inhale deeply for 5-6 minutes.

28. Recipe for Vaginal Dryness

What You Need:
- Bowl for mixing
- Glass jar that seals

Ingredients:
- 2 ounces melted cocoa butter
- 4 ounces parts jojoba oil
- 5 drops sandalwood essential oil
- 2 drops geranium or neroli essential oil

Instructions:
1. Melt the cocoa butter and then add the jojoba oil.
2. Add the essential oils.
3. Warm through and keep stirring to ensure well mixed.
4. Pour into a glass jar and let the mixture to cool. It will solidify.

Twice a day smooth the cream over the tissue using your fingers. You can use just before intercourse too, for more comfortable intercourse.

29. Recipe to Fight Germs

Here is an excellent antiseptic, germ fighting spray that you can use to disinfect your hands, on cuts and scrapes, or to spray a room. It's more effective and safer than many of the commercial products on the market.

What You Need:
- Spray bottle

Ingredients:
- 30 drops tea tree essential oil
- 15 drops eucalyptus essential oil
- 10 drops lemon essential oil
- 8 ounces distilled water

Instructions:
1. Mix all ingredients in your spray bottle.
2. Shake each time before use.

30. Recipe to Stop Snoring

Many snorers have benefited from thyme, while others have found lavender, peppermint, eucalyptus and cypress better. Put the oil on your feet.

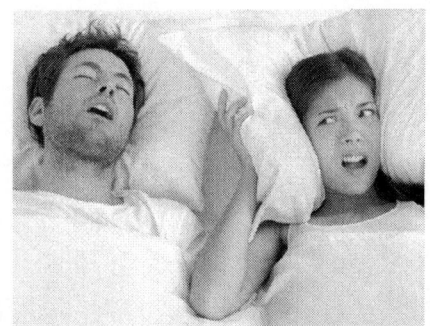

You can also apply it to your nasal region and throat. Experiment which way you get the best results. It's worth it if you can stop snoring.

31. Recipe to Make Your Own "Vapor-Rub"

What You Need:
- Glass jar with a seal
- Saucepan
- Spoon

Ingredients:
- 8 Tbsp. beeswax
- 4 Tbsp. olive oil
- 20 Tbsp. coconut oil
- 40 drops rosemary essential oil
- 20 drops tea tree essential oil

Instructions:
1. Chop up your beeswax.
2. In a saucepan, melt the coconut oil, beeswax and olive oil.
3. Add the essential oils while mixing well.
4. Remove from heat and pour into a glass jar.
5. Let cool and then seal.

32. Recipe for Cough Syrup

Take the warm cough syrup by the spoonful, or if you like, you can mix it with hot water or tea.

When the cough syrup cools, the coconut oil will harden.

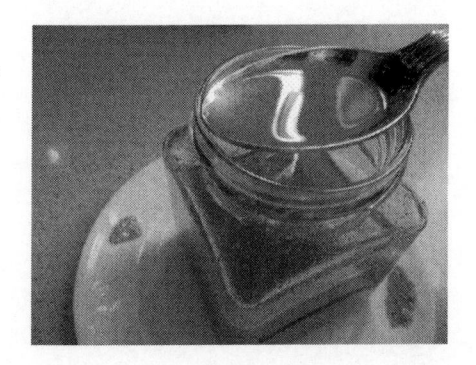

Store it in the refrigerator and when you need to take it, just warm it. It will keep 4-6 weeks.

What You Need:
- Saucepan
- Glass container with lid to store

Ingredients:
- 12 drops of lemon essential oil
- 1 cup local raw honey
- 8 Tbsp. coconut oil

Instructions:
1. Mix all the ingredients together in a saucepan.
2. Heat on low heat until everything is melted. Constantly stir.
3. Pour into glass container and seal.

33. Recipe for Ear Infection

When it comes to ear infection, most doctors still turn to antibiotics to treat. Yet we know that antibiotic use is out of control and there are risks associated with this overuse.

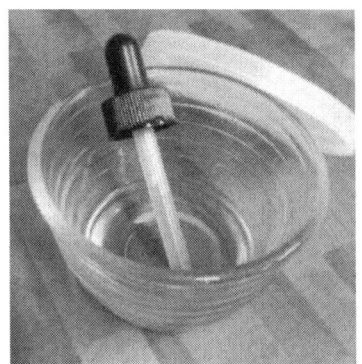

If you or your child has an ear infection, here are some better options to use.

The cotton ball method – Take a couple drops of lavender or tea tree essential oils and put them on a cotton ball.

Take the cotton ball gently place it into your ear. 3-4 times a day, change the cotton ball.

Continue with this treatment until the infection is gone. NEVER put essential oils directly into the ear.

Calendula essential oil - Calendula essential oil will draw out the heat. On the outside of your ear, put one drop of oil and then massaged it into the ear. NEVER put essential oils directly into the ear.

Lemon essential oil – Lemon is good for soothing ear pain from an ear infection. In many cases, this is all that's needed to drain the fluid buildup.

Dilute 2-3 drops of lemon essential oil with an equal amount of coconut oil.
Melt the coconut oil, then mix with the essential oil, and gently rub around the outside of your ear.

Be sure to cover your lymph nodes located on the side of your neck. NEVER put essential oils directly into the ear.

Natural Home Care Recipes

Many are not aware that they can use aromatherapy and essential oil recipes to create natural, chemical free home environment. Doing so, can help to create a more balanced environment and it can help with emotions. What many of us don't think about is the chemicals that we are exposed to everyday and how they affect our bodies and minds negatively.

There isn't a product that you can't make to help you keep your home fresh and clean. Laundry detergent, bleach, window cleaner, general cleaner and the list goes on. In this section, I give you some solid recipes to get you started.

Once you experience a home environment free of chemicals and toxins, you'll be looking to create more safe aromatherapy home care products. There is no shortage of recipes available and this is a great place to start.

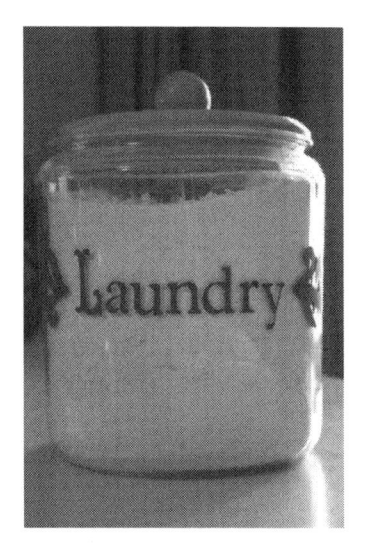

34.   Recipe for Natural Laundry Detergent

What You Need:
- Measuring spoon

- Airtight glass container
- Food processor
- Cheese grater

Ingredients:
- 5 bars (4.5 or 5 oz.) of castile soap
- 3 cups borax
- 5 cups of washing soda
- 45 drops of either lemon or lavender essential oils

Instructions:
1. Grate up all the soap bars
2. Put all of the ingredients in your blender.
3. Blend until the ingredients are well mixed.
4. Store the laundry detergent in an airtight container.

You will need 2-3 tablespoons of detergent per load.

35. Recipe for Homemade Bleach

What You Need:
- A gallon jug

Ingredients:
- Distilled water to fill a gallon jug
- 2 cups lemon juice
- 6 cups 3% hydrogen peroxide
- 25-30 drops lemon essential oil

Instructions:
1. Mix all of the ingredients together into your gallon jug.
2. Gently shake to combine.

Add 1 cup to your washing cycle to whiten and brighten your clothes.

36. Recipe for Citrus All-Purpose Cleaner

What You Need:
- Spray bottle that will hold 8 cups

Ingredients:
- 3cups water
- 3 cups white vinegar
- 30 drops tea tree essential oil
- 15 drops lemon essential oil

Instructions:
1. Place all ingredients into your spray bottle.
2. Shake well before using.

This is an excellent all round cleaning products. DO NOT use on marble.

37. Recipe for Fabric Softener

What You Need:
- A jug

Ingredients:
- 7 cups white vinegar
- ¾ cup rubbing alcohol or you can use vodka
- 40 drops of lavender, tea tree or lemon essential oil

Instructions:
- Put all of the ingredients into your jug.
- Shake it to mix it really well.

Shake before each use. Add ¾ cup in your washing machine's fabric softener dispenser.

38. Recipe to Control Pet Odor

What You Need:
- 8 ounce spray bottle

Ingredients:
- 100 drops lavender essential oil
- 60 drops lemon essential oil
- 30 drops geranium essential oil
- Water

Instructions:
1. Pour the essential oils into your spray bottle.
2. Fill with water.
3. Shake vigorously.

Give it a good shake each time before using. Hold the bottle 12" from your dog, and spray it directly onto your dog. Avoid spraying it near the eyes. You can also spray your dog's bedding, pillow, etc.

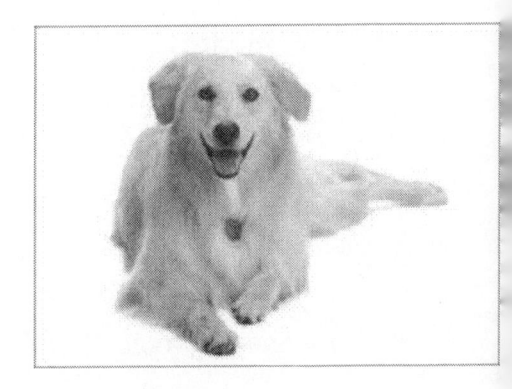

39. Recipe for Glass Cleaner

What You Need:
- Large spray bottle

Ingredients:
- 3 cups water
- 3 cups white vinegar
- ¾ cup rubbing alcohol
- 30 drops lemon essential oil
- 20 drops peppermint essential oil
- 10 drops rosemary essential oil

Instructions:
1. Mix all of the ingredients together in a spray bottle.
2. Shake well.

Before each use, shake well. Spray on glass surfaces and immediately wipe using a clean cloth.

40. Recipe for Dish Soap

What You Need:
- 32 ounce squirt bottle

Ingredients:
- Liquid castile soap
- 20 drops lemon essential oil
- 10 drops orange essential oil

Instructions:
1. Fill the bottle with liquid soap.
2. Add your essential oils.

Before using, shake well.

This is NOT for use in a dishwasher.

Conclusion

If you are here, it means you have made it to the end of the book. That's terrific! I hope you have tried at least some of the recipes and that you keep experimenting and trying the ones you have not yet made.

Aromatherapy is a great way to lift your spirits, help put you in a good mood and balance your emotions. It also plays a key role in helping if you are dealing with pain.

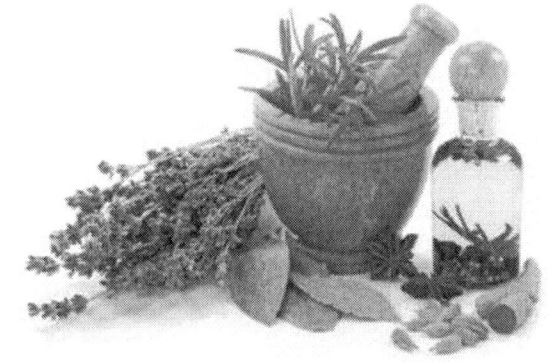

Start to build up a collection of the main essential oils that these recipes use, such as peppermint, lavender or tea tree. Then you'll have them on hand.

I want you to have as many options as possible for products you can make, so that you can match them with your healthy lifestyle.

I know it can be extremely frustrating to buy products that contain all kinds of terrible chemicals. Often, you only seeing the 'tip of the iceburg' as it can be decades later before associations are made between specific ingredients and serious health issues like cancer.

Good news – you never have to do it again! These top 40 aromatherapy recipes are an excellent start. Feel free to make changes to any of these recipes and don't forget to have some fun.

Aromatherapy is an amazing addition to a healthy lifestyle. Having control over what you put on your body and use in your home is empowering. I hope you've enjoyed this book and hope you continue to create your own natural essential oil products.

Printed in Great Britain
by Amazon